CLASSICAL DANCES

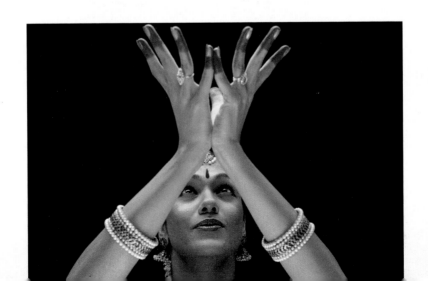

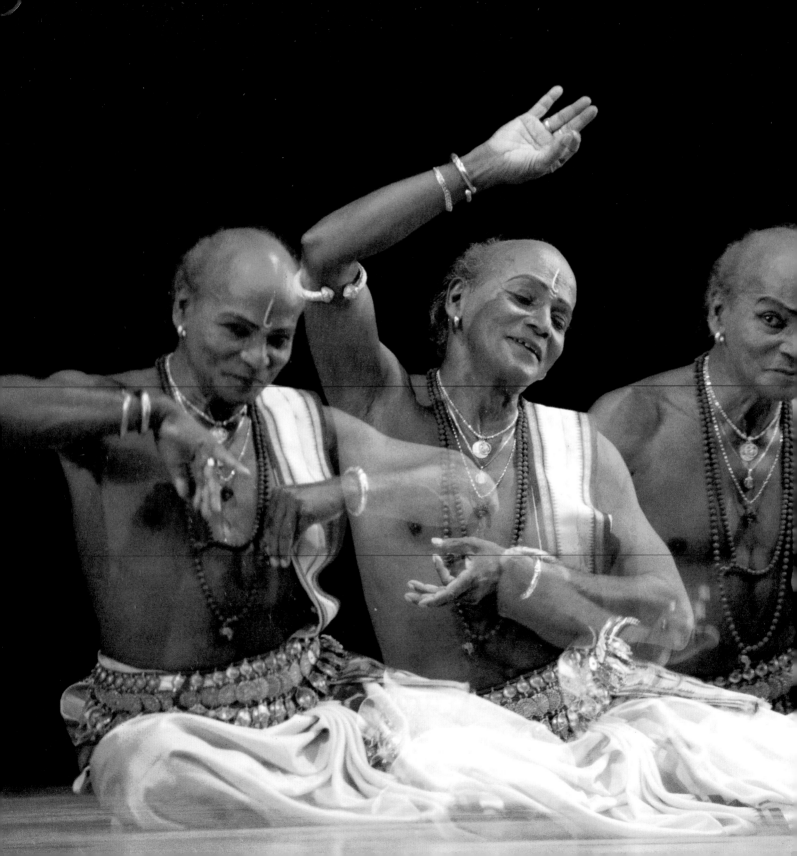

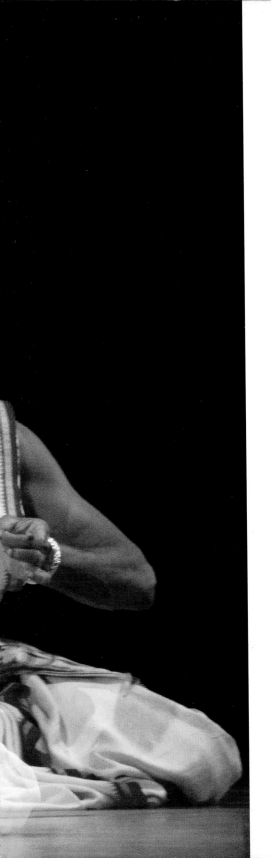

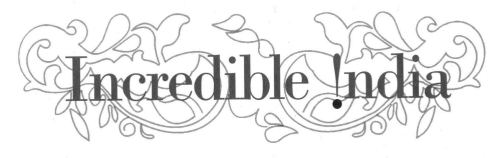

CLASSICAL DANCES

Text Sonal Mansingh
Photographs Avinash Pasricha

wisdom
tree
ACADEMIC

By arrangement with
Department of Tourism, Ministry of Culture, Government of India

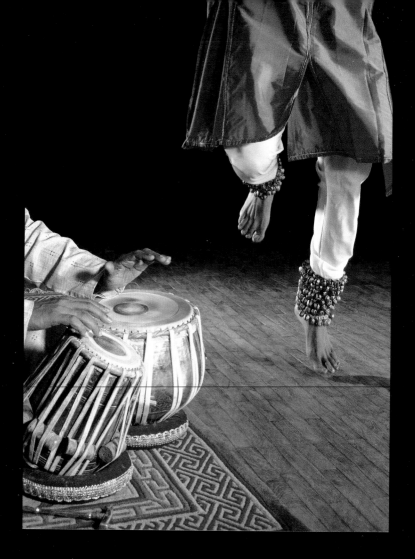

Published in 2007 by

Wisdom Tree
4779/23 Ansari Road, Darya Ganj, New Delhi-110002
Ph: 23247966/67/68

Text © Sonal Mansingh
Photographs © Avinash Pasricha

ISBN   81-8328-067-6

Conceptualised and published by Shobit Arya for Wisdom Tree; *edited by* Manju Gupta; *designed
at* SN Graphix and *printed at* Print Perfect, New Delhi - 110064

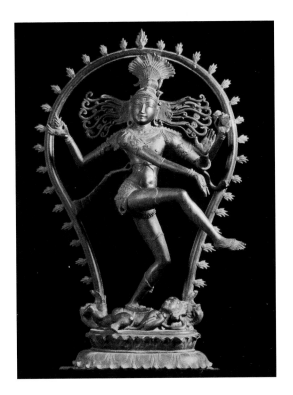

Preface

Combining every aspect of the Indian theory of creation, the figure of Nataraja, as envisioned by sages and seers in their deepest meditations, has withstood the testimony of time, millennia after millennia. The dark unknown mass, now discovered by astrophysicists and scientists, was known to India as *Shiva* (that which is auspicious and exudes beatitude) or as *purusha* (that which was before everything). Charged by vibrations which arise, just as a desire arises in the heart and activates a person to act, in the mass or matter, Shiva was galvanised, forming innumerable atoms of creation in a process which is still on and promises to continue for an unknown number of time-cycles yet to come. We have now learnt through intricate calculations of great minds that space is elastic, ever expanding, limitless, and in this space swim innumerable galaxies, each containing millions of solar systems, stars, milky ways and black holes.

Such a mystically majestic discovery is not a gift of our own 20th-21st century only. This was known to Indians early enough who, instead of confining such a vast vision only to science and mathematics, gave it a poetic metaphor and thus was born the concept of Shiva Nataraja.

Once the dark unknown mass which emits no light but is the cause for creation to come into being was transferred to metaphorical realms, there was no looking back. Every known natural and scientific process was represented as attributed in this metaphor. This is how one has to look at the figure of Shiva Nataraja to comprehend the exact moment of creation, the Big Bang.

Four arms show the superhuman status as also indicate the engulfing of the four directions. The left upper arm holds fire, symbolising light. This is the light of knowledge which helps in God-realisation. The right upper arm holds a small *damaru* (drum), signifying those subtle vibrations of sound that are at the root of every form in creation. The left lower arm is thrown across his torso towards right and points downwards at the uplifted left leg, indicating elevation of all beings from their mundane existence. The right lower arm rests on the left in a gesture of *abhaya* (fear not). It is both a benediction and a promise. The right foot is firmly planted on the back of a gnarled and twisted figure of a dwarf, who is *apasmara* – a symbol of darkness, ignorance and arrogance. River Ganga flows out of Shiva's flying hair. The root of the name 'Ganga' is '*gam*', meaning 'to go', 'to flow'. Therefore, everything which is in the form of a flow is called Ganga, including the flow of life. A crescent moon like a thin silvery sliver shines on his forehead. This is the moon on the second day of the bright fortnight signifying a continuous play of waxing and waning in creation. He is draped in a tiger skin to show his victory over every ferocious and fearsome element. Viewed from behind, a bronze statue of Shiva Nataraja demonstrates a supple serpentine spine with the body perfectly balanced on the right foot. The plumb-line of the body from head to toe is absolutely straight. The aura of fire around the figure is the manifested creation which comes into being as his dance progresses. This is the moment of cosmic creation.

- Sonal Mansingh

Contents

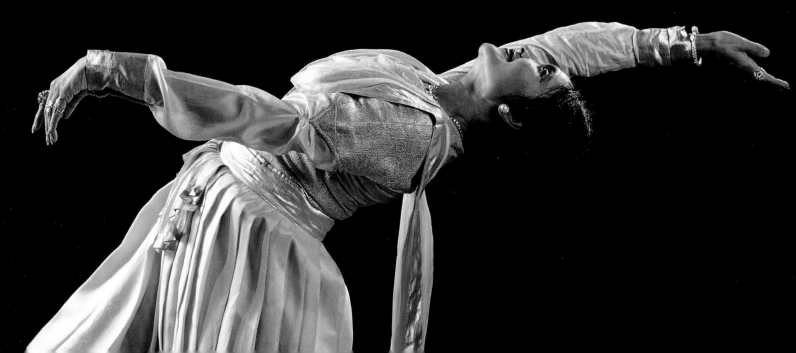

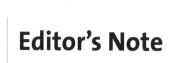

Editor's Note

India, home to one of the most ancient civilisations, is a unique example of cultural and geographical diversities. Dissimilar cultural practices are deeply rooted in people's daily lives even in the 21st century. Indian history is the fruit of geography, and geography the root of history. The history of several millennia has merged with phenomenal geographical variations to create the incredible India of today.

India is incredible in its landscapes, and the people who adorn her. Its rituals and traditions; sculptures and paintings; dance, music and theatre; handicrafts, fairs and festivals; monuments and manuscripts; and its varied cuisine – each is a definite statement that only India can proudly pronounce.

Myriad streams and rivers have been flowing for centuries in their own special terrain, sometimes forceful, sometimes gentle. Despite all kinds of obstacles, they flow on. When these waters reach the ocean, they mingle, and become one huge ocean. Similarly, these diverse, astonishingly rich and colourful cultural currents create a harmonious hymn known as India, even as they retain their unique individual identity.

This series of Incredible India presents 10 books on different cultural aspects of the country, written by well-known experts on the subject. This book on Indian classical dance has been written by one of India's finest danseuse. As she traces dancing figures in ancient civilisation, describes dancers from the *Vedas*, narrates various interpretations of the cosmic dance of Shiva Nataraj she covers the span of 5,000 years. For those who are involved in classical dance, music and theatre the famous treatise of Bharata known as *Bharata Natya Shastra* is an important point of reference. For Sonal Mansingh it is a milestone on highway.

The author, herself being an exponent of Bharatanatyam and Odissi, has described Bharatanatyam of the south quite at length. After that she covers Odissi from Orissa, Kathak from the North, Kathakali and Mohiniattam from Kerala, Manipuri from Manipur, Kuchipudi from Andhra Pradesh, and Sattriya from Assam. Talking about any Indian art is never complete without touching upon its interconnectedness with other art forms. It is fortunately so because that denotes Indian-ness to the art, even when it is taken up individually. This book is enriched with the author's personal anecdotes.

Avinash Pasricha has a treasure-trove of photographs so far as dancers and musicians are concerned. He has been capturing them in his camera from various angles, in different moods and costumes, at all kinds of locales, be it at the seashore, inside or outside a temple or in an air-conditioned auditorium!

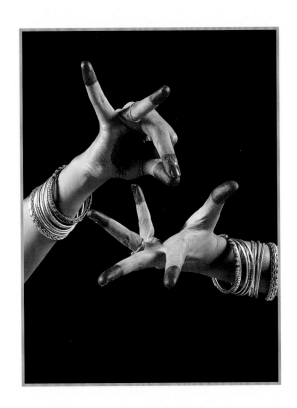

Concept of Dance in India

In a land touching the Himalayan heights and reaching down to the south where three oceans meet, from the lush green eastern boundary with Myanmar and China to the deserts of Rajasthan and Gujarat bordering Pakistan in the west, India harbours a staggering variety of cultures and sub-cultures. With teeming millions of people who follow numerous religions and social beliefs, speak many languages and dialects, practice a bewildering array of customs and manners, the wonder remains — the wonder of those commonly shared pan-Indian attitudes, mores and beliefs that cut through deep ravines and high mountains, thick forests, sandy wilderness and gushing but unpredictable rivers. Legends and myths that have endured through millennia and are still active in various strata of society have held this astonishing multiplicity together. In the Indic tradition, myths are not just fairy-tales. Legends and myths are based on real events. These are called *Puranas* in Sanskrit, meaning 'that which happened a long time ago but has been stored in collective memory of many generations'. Thus began the two systems of accruing knowledge — *shruti*, that which is heard, and *smruti*, that which is stored in memory.

A student or seeker stores up the lessons, observations, experiences, names, ideas and their contexts in his memory. At an exact moment the information is summoned and it flows out smoothly, having marinated and matured in the meanwhile. *Shruti* insists on concentrated listening by a routinely lazy or mindless ear because otherwise it can never receive and convey the exact phase or word to the mind. Given the nuances, diction and pronunciation of letters in Sanskrit and many other Indian languages, a student is supposed to be an attentive and perfect listener. In the second phase, the word and its meaning is carried to the mind's storage bin and placed in the appropriate slot. At a signal, the slot opens to allow the relevant information/knowledge/recitation/context to tumble out. This is *smruti*. Indian dance works on the assumption of further exploration and enhancement of any given idea. Cutting across geographical, social, religious and linguistic barriers, the ideas, images and legends have endured to form a pool of water in which every dancer is baptised, regardless of the style of dance she/he pursues.

For a quick glance through the kaleidoscope of commonly found names, ideas and metaphors, let us first consider the long list of names of divinities who inhabit the common spaces in philosophical, religious, social and art traditions. To begin from the beginning, the first sound is *aum*. The three letters are supposed to denote the three qualities or *guna* (in creation), namely *sattva* (pure), *rajas* (self-conscious) and *tamas* (dark, hidden) or the three tenses or *trikaala*, viz, *bhuta* (past), *vartaman* (present) and *bhavishya* (future) or the three levels, viz. *akaash* (heaven), *prithvi* (earth) and *pataal* (netherworld). The sound itself is called the life-breath of creation and is the first manifestation of energy waves which vibrate and galvanise all inert matter. Because energy waves emanate from one centre, the point of balance between unmanifested and manifested creation, it is called Brahman, meaning 'the vast expanse'. Thus Indian thought begins with *aum* and is carried to the ordinary man through dance and music to become an integral part of the ethos of dance.

The different aspects of creation (energy) are given different names which are derived from their role in maintaining the life cycle on earth and the cycles of the ever-expanding and contracting universe. This has also been the case of every ancient civilisation. God is called *agni* to signify a blazing fire in the form of the Sun, hunger in the stomach, fury in temperament, sexual desire and worldly ambitions. Prefixes are added to distinguish one form of fire from the other. A dancer should be able to delineate *kamagni*, the fire of sexual desire, from *jatharagni*, the fire of hunger through her delineation. Yet the god of fire, Agni's icon, remains constant where he is shown possessing seven tongues symbolising seven flames with the aggressive ram as his vehicle. Similarly the gods of wind, rain, thunderstorm and water, each with their own weapons, vehicles and

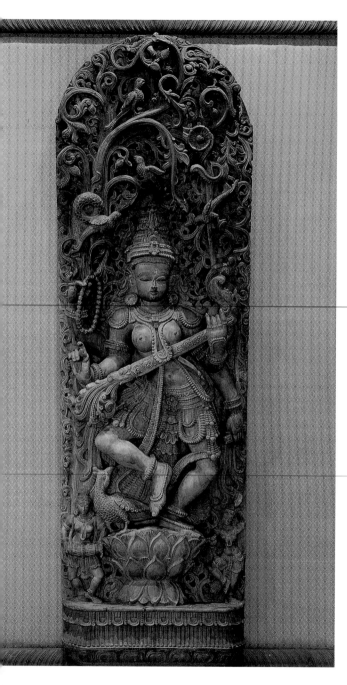

consorts are common motifs in dance and sculptures. There is Saraswati, the goddess of learning and knowledge, who holds a beautifully-carved stringed instrument called the *veena*, showing her as a patron of music and every other art form. Her vehicle is a white swan which conveys purity of the soul. The goddess of wealth is Lakshmi, wherein the root word, *lakshm* meaning 'restless' is worshipped and requested to stay put in a household or business, so that she does not vanish. Stories of sisterhood and sibling rivalry are favourite themes with dancers. There are many stories of billionaires and kings turning penniless overnight for not respecting the presence of Lakshmi. Further, there are presiding deities for every direction and angle, for every hour of day and night, for every element in Nature to convey to the egoistic human the importance of humility and consideration towards everything around. In the hierarchy of divine beings, those who are in the highest realm are Devi, Shiva, Vishnu, Krishna and Ganesha.

The Indian dancer is at once a scholar, linguist, philosopher, musician and believer. If the dancer does not know or understand the meanings of names, their symbolism and iconography, their connection and context to each other and to the world of humans and the wider cosmos, then she/he is unable to convey the essential flavour and meaning of the concept.

Devi: Derived from the root *div* in Sanskrit, it means 'light'; thus Devi means 'the great goddess who illumines and energises creation'. She has millions of forms and attributes, names and legends, because she is manifested in every atom in space. Some of the oft-used names are Jagadamba or mother of the constant flux of creation and destruction; Bhavani, who is the cause of all happenings; Kali, the dark one; Gauri the

LEFT
Saraswati, Goddess of Learning, Arts and Refinements, playing on the veena, *the ancient string instrument, in a dance posture*

fair one; and Mahishasur Mardini, slayer of sloth, ignorance and demonic forces. She appears as Parvati, the daughter of the king of Himalayas and is married to Shiva, the great god. In other words, she is simply Amba (mother) having two sons, Ganesha and Kartikeya.

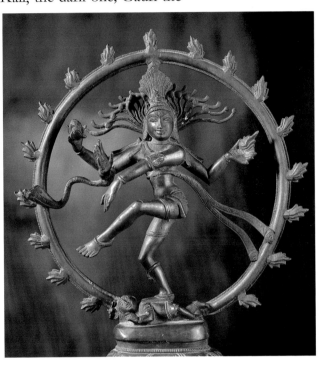

Shiva: In the anthropomorphic form of *linga*, Shiva is worshipped as the *axis mundi* spanning heaven but rooted in earth; as Nataraja, the king of dancers, he is seen in his dynamic form; as Dakshinamurti, he is the guru, the teacher; as Bhairav he is fearsome; as Rudra, he is the ferocious one; as Sundareshwar, he is the most handsome; and as Vishwanath, he is the lord of the universe.

For every weapon held in his four or more arms and for every demon slain he assumes a new name which the dancer employs in his/her story to emphasise a special mood. Interestingly, Shiva literally means 'beatific and auspicious'.

Vishnu: He is the one that sustains the creation. Giving recognisable form

ABOVE
Shiva, the Supreme Dancer. This iconic image conceives of the moment of Creation as Shiva dances, uplifting the universe with the left upraised leg while trampling down on ignorance

to the concept has created so many personas that the dancer finds himself/herself veritably in a crowd of identities with whom he/she converses and interacts. It is this internalised dialogue with a name or a form behind a concept that the dancer depicts. Some of the popular aspects of Vishnu are: *anantshayin*, i.e. resting on 'timeless time' and shown as a giant serpent/cobra floating on a milky ocean — *ksheer sagara shyama*, because milk symbolises sustenance and nourishment. Vishnu as Lakshmi's husband is called Lakshminarayan and Vishnu alone as Narayana — he who is within and around. One of the abiding myths is about the 10 incarnations of Vishnu called the *Dashaavatara*. The theme speaks about recurring periods of evil perpetuated by arrogant and violent demons or anti-gods and the necessity of Vishnu arriving on the scene to remove or annihilate them and set the cosmic balance right again.

They are:

matsya	-	fish
koorma	-	tortoise
varaha	-	wild boar
narasimha	-	man-lion
varmana	-	midget
Parasurama	-	warrior Brahmin
Rama	-	king or chieftain
Krishna	-	dark one
Balarama	-	tiller or agriculturist
kalki	-	end of an aeonic cycle

An intelligent dancer connects this to the process of evolution as can be seen from the first incarnation which occurs in elemental waters; the second equally in water and on land; the third being wild boar digging deep into the earth; fourth shows half entry of human and of animal species; and the fifth brings the early man as short in physical stature. The conflicts and struggles

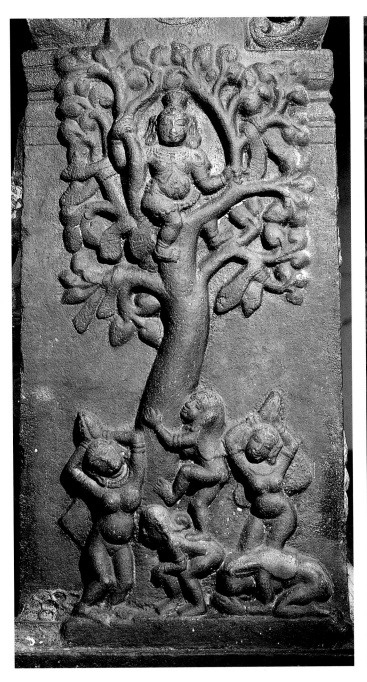
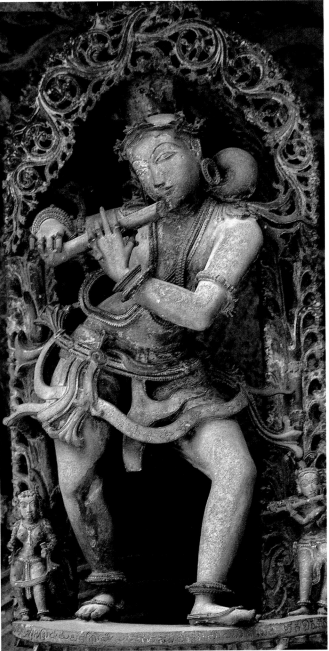

of earlier times are depicted by the sixth and subsequently, the settled security of a ruler gives us the seventh: the eighth incarnation, Krishna, has been seen as a 'synonym for Vishnu himself' taking the human form with the totality of every attribute he possesses. In settled times, agriculture flourished and is shown in the ninth incarnation. According to every known school and sect of Vaishnavism, the above nine incarnations have already taken place in our aeonic time or cycle. The tenth and the last one to arrive on the scene will be Kalki, who is described as a ball of fire riding on a white horse and holding a sharp sword drawn. He would bring this aeonic drama to a close for a new one to begin, after Creation has rested a while as seen in the image of Vishnu resting on the serpent or as an *ananta*, i.e. without an end.

Krishna: The dark, handsome, mischievous, charismatic, romantic hero of the epic *Mahabharata* and the philosophical *Bhagawad Gita*. Krishna occupies a very special place in the Indian mind. His stormy childhood when he kills innumerable demonic forces, his romantic love for the milkmaids of Vraja, his naughty pranks in stealing butter and milk, his special relationship with Radha — all have given dance material to dancers of all ages and practice. His flute-playing, his special attire of a peacock feather tucked in his hair and a striking yellow cloth draped around the dark swarthy body have provided rich imagery for poets, sculptors, painters and dancers. An inexplicable fascination with this mysterious figure persists among the country-folk and urban dwellers alike. Among the many names by which he is called are included Madhava (sweet as honey), Keshava (of thick, curly, unruly hair), Govinda (knower of the illumined self), Gopal (protector of light shown in the symbol of a cow), Vanamali (wearer of a garland of jungle flowers), Ghanashyam (dark as the rain-bearing clouds), Hari (who removes sorrow and pain), Giridhari (one who lifts Mount Govardhana). Endlessly the dancers of every dance form portray one or more of the

PAGE 15 LEFT
Krishna as the stealer of human ego which gives illusory sense of self-importance and vanity

PAGE 15 RIGHT
Krishna adopted the flute as his instrument for spreading the message of love. Melodies emanating from his venu *(flute) bewitched humans, birds and beasts alike*

countless episodes and stories from his life as recorded in the *Srimad Bhagawad* and many other texts.

Ganesha: This is a god with the head of an elephant to symbolise wisdom and capacity to remove and overcome any obstacle. Ganesha is the son of Parvati, the adoring mother, and an indulgent Shiva, the father. Ganesha is often portrayed as a baby seated on Parvati's lap with a round ball of sweet in his pudgy hand. He has a portly stomach to contain the secrets of creation, hence the name Lambodara. For his elephant-shaped head, he is called Gajanana and because he blesses the devotees by removing obstacles and troubles, he is called Vighna Vinayaka. He is also shown dancing in a variety of postures as Nritya Vinayaka, and as the chief of Shiva's motley group of *gana* (goblins), he is Ganesha. All such images and iconographies are woven into dance, usually in a dance or music performance and even in traditional theatre forms of India. An invocation is offered to Ganesha at the beginning of every performance to seek his blessings for a smooth presentation.

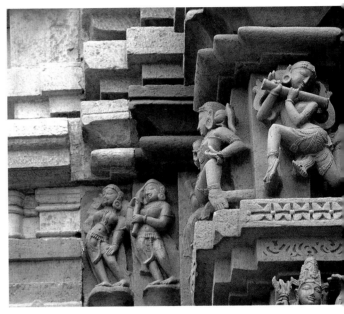

Some of the more popular themes basic to all dance styles are the *navarasa* and the *ashtanayika*. *Navarasa* refers to the classification of human emotions under nine heads. *Rasa* is one of the two key words of Indian aesthetics, the other being *ananda*. *Rasa* has been loosely translated as flavour, juice, essence, emotion, sentiment and mood. The totality of any experience reviewed and recalled in repose can give the kind of pleasure and delight which immediacy of the same experience may not have given at the moment of its happening. This kind of pleasure translates into *rasa*, rather,

ABOVE
A flute player on the temple-wall accompanying the dancer in the adjoining niche

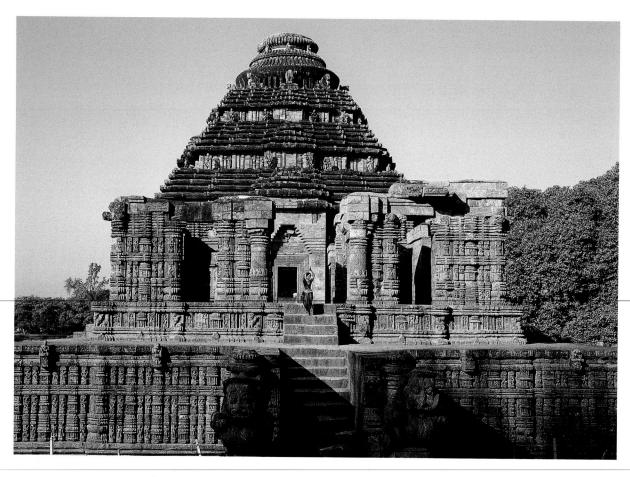

the taste of *rasa*, the aesthetic delight. By observation and experience, eight categories were classified to understand and successfully portray human emotions. These are described and explained in great detail by Bharata in his classic compendium on theatre, the *Natya Shastra*. The eight moods are of *sringara* (love), *veer* (valour), *karun* (pathos), *hasya* (mirth), *raudra* (furious), *adbhut* (wonder), *bhaya* (fearful) and *bibhatsa* (disdainful). The ninth of the present-day *navarasas* is the mood of *shanta* (tranquillity), which was added to the list in the 11th century.

A detailed depiction of the *navarasa* contained in poems relating to *Ramayana*, Devi or Krishna episodes are popular with every dancer. Another abiding motif is that of the *nayika*, the romantic heroine. Indian aesthetics give great importance to the idea of romantic love by laying emphasis on the types of hero and heroine, their temperament, age, experience, appearance, etc. The *sringara rasa* has the distinction of being given the title of *Adi Rasa* (the first and origin of emotions) and *rasaraj* (king of *rasa*). *Sringara* or love rules our lives. Love in any form and relationship exists in Nature as in humans. The mutual attraction and distraction, the romantic tension between sexes, the ensuing body language and voluntary or involuntary reactions naturally form the basis on which the idea of *ashtanayika* is anchored. They are:

Abhisarika	-	leaving home to meet lover
Vasakasajja	-	fully adorned and prepared
Virahotkanthita	-	unable to bear separation
Vipralabdha	-	disappointed, deceived
Khardita	-	angry, jealous
Kalahantarita	-	repentant after the quarrel
Proshitpatika	-	waiting for him who has gone abroad
Swadheenbhartika	-	adored by the lover

The classification according to age shows a young woman, almost adolescent, on the threshold of life making her first shy, hesitant entry into the world of love. She is called *mugdha*. The woman, who, having experienced romantic love, is sure of her hold on the lover is called *pragalbha*. And in advancing age, she who still wields mature charm is called *praudha*. Then there are those who show their upbringing and station in life by their belligerent and unbridled temperament. They are *adhama*, the lowest. One who knows the pitfalls of losing control either in anger or jealousy, yet occasionally falls prey to it is *madhyama*, the middling. She who exercises

LEFT
Konark, the temple dedicated to Surya, the sun. Situated on the eastern seashore, the walls and lintels of the main temple and those of the natya mandap *i.e. dance-hall are replete with carved images of dancers, musicians, lovers, flora and fauna*

great control over passion and temper and is ever smiling and pleasant, is called *uttama*, the best.

This and much more go into the building up of a dancer's training to a point when situations, stories and characters do not remain strange but become an intimate part of her inner world. Then, without the aid of props, special lights, and technology, she creates a world of magical happenings and characters. Using the power of transforming mundane happenings and situations into extraordinary and describing the art, the Indian dancer today is adept at comprehending contemporary issues like environmental degradation, ecological balance, women's rights, human rights, child abuse, world peace, problems of survival in a mechanised society and much more. The rich and varied vocabulary of dance becomes a handy tool to pinpoint these without becoming banal and pedestrian.

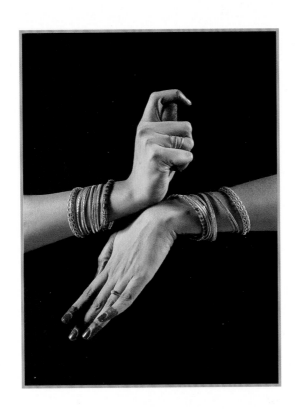

Bharatanatyam

The term 'Bharatanatyam' has two connotations — first, Bharata is considered to be the name of a sage-scholar to whom is attributed the first comprehensive treatise on theatre, music and dance, called the *Natya Shastra*; the second connotation breaks up the word *Bharata* into three syllables: *bha* for *bhava* (emotion), *ra* for *raga* (music) and *ta* for *tala* (rhythm). The term *natyam* implies theatre, though today the term signifies a classical dance system that has made the southern states of Tamil Nadu and Karnataka its home. In the 17th, 18th, and 19th centuries, this dance was also known as Sadir, Nautch or Dasiattam. The origins, as with other classical styles, are in the time-honoured traditions systematised and codified by Bharata. This dance form consists of *nritta* and *nritya*, meaning 'pure dance' and 'narrational dance'. Let us consider the components of each separately, beginning with *nritta*.

PAGE 21
'Parrot perched on a branch'

RIGHT
'Dreaming while asleep' — the import of a song about a young woman's unrequited love and intense longing for the beloved has been a favourite theme. The love of a woman for her loved one gets translated to the other level where the soul yearns to be reunited with the One
- T. Balasaraswati

Bharatanatyam begins with a salutation to the guru, taking the first steps in pure dance or *nritta*. Initially the basic posture — *aramandi* (also called *ardhamandali*) has to be mastered before the initiate can even lift a foot. This posture shows the legs bent at the knee, the knees turned out, the feet turned out joining at the heels, stomach held in, hands placed neatly on the hips and the torso inclining forward slightly. From this posture emanates the entire corpus of *adavus* (units of dance), beginning with the simple exercise of lifting the right foot up to the level of the other knee and beating it down forcefully on the ground to produce a clap-like sound. This is repeated with the left foot and, alternately, the feet rise and fall in three variations of tempo — slow, medium and fast, bearing in mind that only the legs move without any supporting movement of the torso, hands or the head.

PAGE 24
Grace of body and clean lines predominate Bharatanatyam - Alarmel Valli

The moment the right leg is extended sideways, resting on the heel, the right arm, which is held aloft, slightly bent at the elbow with the hand in the *tripataka* gesture (outstretched palm with the third finger bent) twisted, making the arm straight, palm facing upwards, the head turns to the right, looking at the hand.

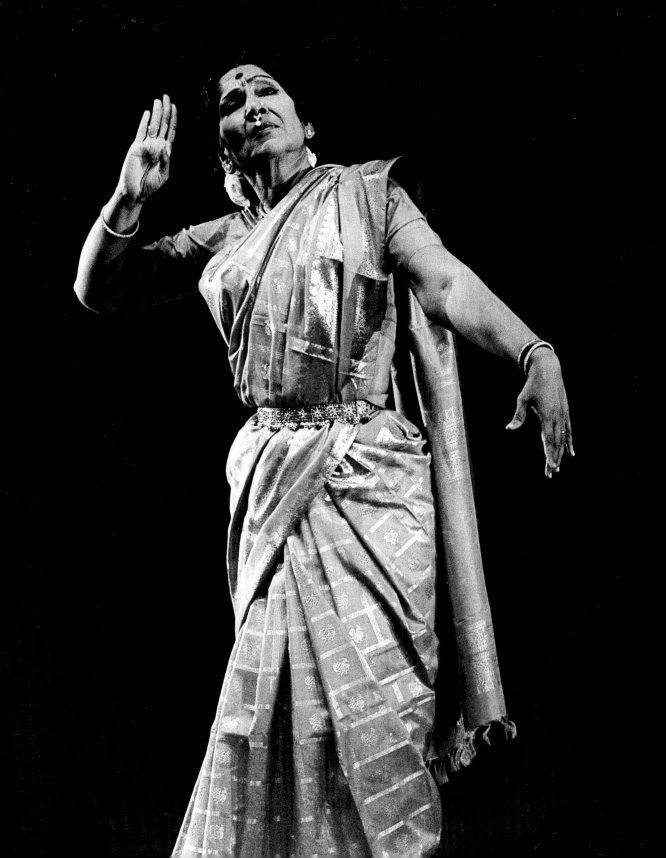

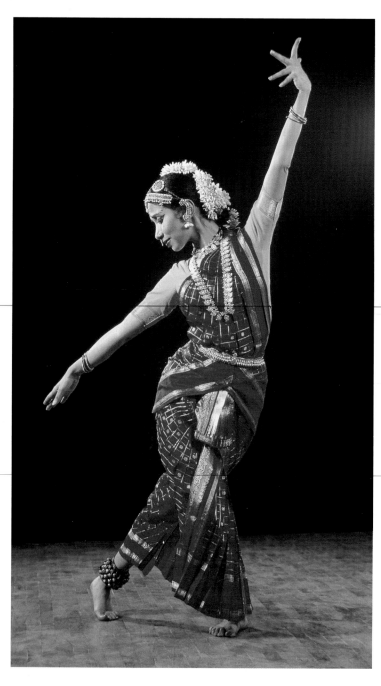

The second phase of this *adavu* consists of bringing back the outstretched leg to its original position, while simultaneously turning the palm outwards (facing the front) and the arm assuming the semi-circular position, with the head brought to its initial position, looking straight. The same movement is repeated on the left side.

Once the student masters the co-ordination of movements, he/she moves forward to complicated patterns involving flat-footed stamps, jumps on toes, beating of the foot in toe-heel combinations, sitting on toes and then leaping up like a released spring and movements, circular or lateral, with arms held above the head or outstretched at the chest, weaving a design of crisscross squares and triangles while the hands fold and unfold in flower-like movements to make different *hasta* (hand gestures used in pure dance). Bharatanatyam revels in neatness of line which gives the pure dance a geometrical majesty comparable to the architectural grandeur of the south Indian temples. There are nine groups of *adavu*s — each group consisting of three or more variations which become successively complicated in execution.

There are a set of exercises for the concerned limbs — the feet, ankles, knees, waist, torso, shoulders, wrists, fingers and head to tune the body before physical and visual music of dance can be produced.

The next stage includes a unit of successive *adavu*s with a *teermanam* (rounding off) called the *jati*. Then follows the dance proper, called *alarippu*. This is the shortest dance in the repertoire and is designed to set up the technical framework which provides a base for the succeeding items. It involves movements of the eyes and eyebrows, along with the sideways, gliding neck movements termed *attami* in Tamil and *sundari* (*rechaka*) in Sanskrit; movements which the student has learned at the time of practicing the *adavu*s. Proceeding from the eyes and neck, with feet together, knees straight, the body erect and the balance distributed equally on both legs, the shoulders and hands standing erect in *samapada* are moved in smooth glides and jerks, moving sideways and front. The process is repeated in the fully seated posture, which leads to the other half of the dance, where slightly more complicated locomotion, footwork, bends and hand

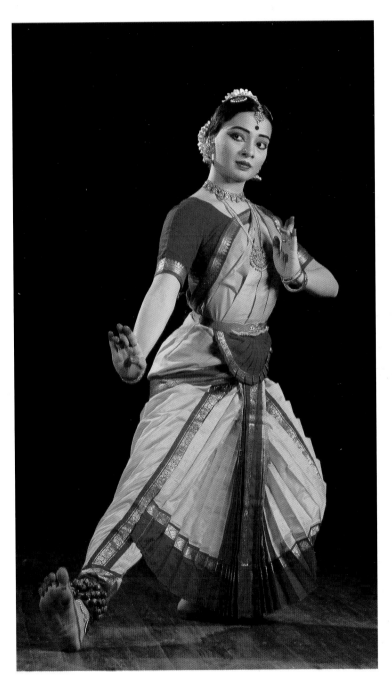

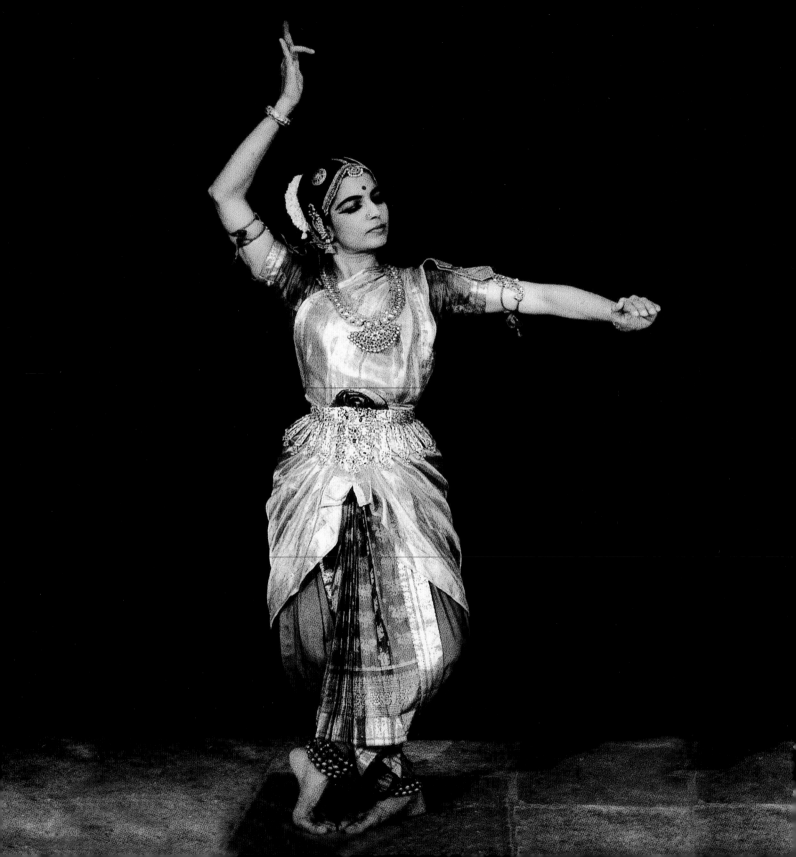

gestures build up to the flourish of a short *jati*, to bring the dance to a close. The garland-like movements of the arms give it the character of a greeting and salutation.

Now comes the more complicated dance patterns and rhythms of the *jatiswaram*, the second step in the repertoire. The name itself suggests the character of the dance — a string of *jatis* set to the *swarams* or musical notations of a particular melodic mode, the *raga*. The *alarippu* is danced to rhythmic syllables uttered by the teacher, reproduced on the cymbals and percussion instruments; it is thus unaccompanied by any song as such. The second element, *nritya*, is the next item. Great literary works set to music are introduced at this stage and these are to be translated in dance through the medium of *nritya-abhinaya*, the evocative communication, in which playing with subtle nuances and suggestive gestures, laying bare the soul of the theme contained in the relevant song, are the defining characteristics.

The student now proceeds to manipulate the 10 fingers separately or together to produce a myriad images, which infuse colour into the words of a song, vivifying the situations and characters. According to Bharata, there are 24 gestures through the use of both hands and 28 with one hand. The technical terms for these are *samyukta hasta* and *asamyukta hasta*. *Hasta* means 'hand' in Sanskrit. Each *hasta* has a name which either refers to the literal meaning of the word or simply describes the mechanics of arriving at the gesture. For example, the hand gesture called *allapadma* means 'a full-blown lotus'. The gesture itself resembles a lotus flower in which the fingers are outstretched from a curved palm to look like the petals of a lotus. Here the Sanskrit term, its literal meaning and the hand gesture combine together to create a total image. There are others, like the *tripataka*, which is a method of forming the hand gesture, *tri* meaning 'third' and *pataka* meaning 'the flag' which is the first gesture of the series. Thus, by bending the third finger into the *pataka* gesture, one arrives at the *tripataka*. Among the double hand gestures, the most easily recognisable is *anjali* or 'an offering or obeisance'.

PAGE 25
Geometry of parallel or diagonal lines, triangles and squares is an integral and significant part of the technique
- Malavika Sarukkai

LEFT
Dancing entire stories of legends and episodes through judicious use of hand-gestures (mudra), body-postures and facial expressions constitute the second element, integral to Bharatanatyam
- Rukmini Devi

It is performed by joining both the palms of the hands in a typical Indian salutation called *namaskar*, *namaste* or *pranam*.

Each gesture can denote or connote objects and ideas. To illustrate this, let us consider the *allpadma* gesture which has the possibilities of showing the lotus, a flower, a full moon, the sun, a place, a mountain, a beautiful face, the bosom, an elaborate hairdo, etc. These are all recognisable. The same hand gestures can now be used to show beauty and oneself — questioning, mockery, dalliance. The treatise and commentaries like *Abhinaya Darpana* (Mirror of Gestures) by Nandi Keshwara list many usages, hinting that a dancer is at liberty to use her skill and intelligence in creating new connotations.

Hands are not alone in their quest for expression. The face, specially the eyes, play an equally important role, sometimes even rendering the use of hand gestures unnecessary. Each component of the face is brought into play, but before one can gain a mastery over their use, their direction and movements are essential. The eyebrows have to move separately or together — up and down, quivering or knitted. The eyes are mirrors of the soul, a man's searchlight spanning the three worlds.

Eyes that encompass spheres, directions and emotions, indeed are creations. The shape of the eye has been compared to a lotus petal of a fish; the glance to a gazelle or as hypnotic as a cobra's. Indian classical literature is full of allusions about the beauty and propensity of eyes. Thus, it is not surprising that Indian dance has also laid so much emphasis on *drishti* (glance, the look). To be able to convey emotions — subtle or gross, the eyes must be trained to move vertically, horizontally, in half or full circle, zig-zag or slantwise, with the pupils dilated or contracted. To facilitate a clear movement, the eyes are opened twice the normal size by pushing the upper eyelids upwards with the index finger and the lower still lower with the thumb while doing the exercises. This also strengthens the eye muscles which might explain the comparative absence of bespectacled dancers.

RIGHT
Lotus-hands, front knee bend, both feet aligned in a straight line and looking at the outstretched parallel lines of arm and leg completes a complex dance pattern called adavu
-Priyadarshini Govind

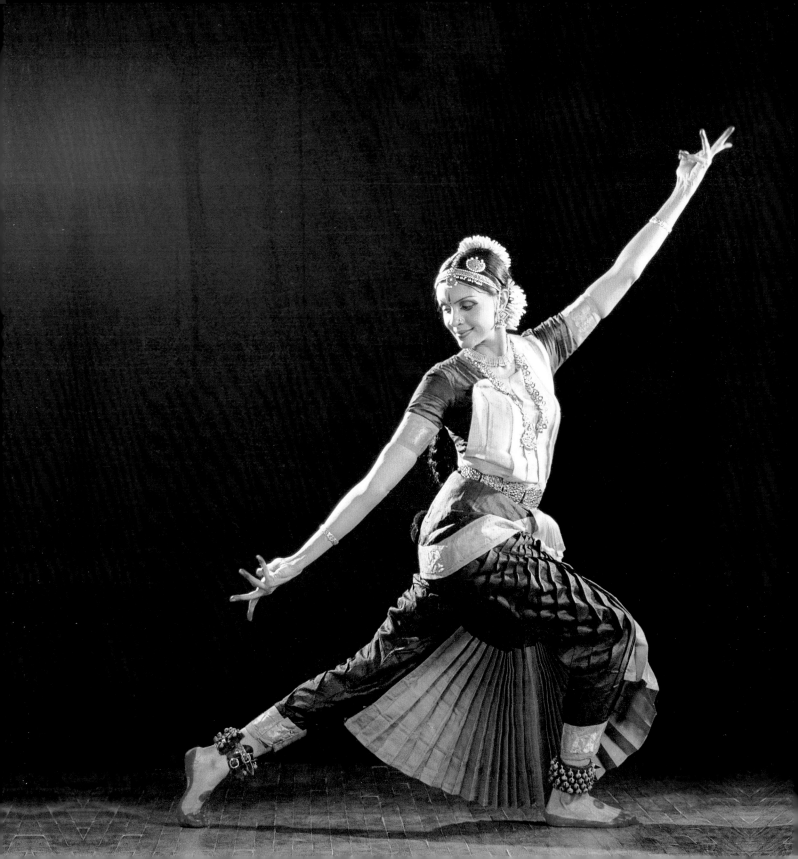

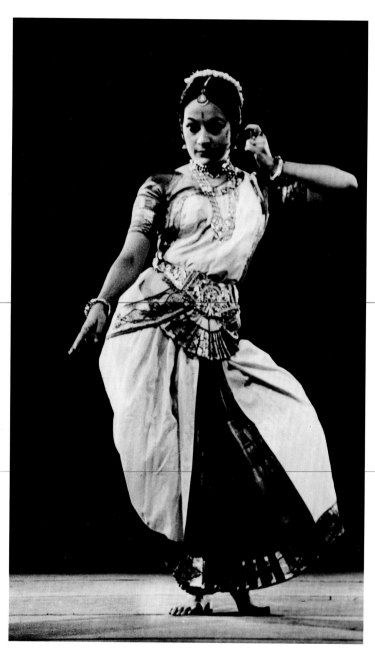

Great dancers have been known to perform *abhinaya* for a considerable length of time purely with their eyes — summoning, rejecting, yearning, mocking or beseeching. The ancient verse which I quote below sums up the concept of aesthetics of movement and expression very aptly: *yato hastaha*, which means where the hand goes the glance follows; where the eyes go, the mind follows; where the mind is involved, emotions arise; and where emotions ripple, *rasa* (flavour) permeates the work of art.

The nostrils are capable of showing happiness and sadness by looking pinched or dilated. The mouth is capable of remaining natural, pursed to show displeasure, drooping downwards to express contempt and mockery, slightly open to show surprise, and extended to express joy, mirth and happiness. The neck, which has been compared to a lotus stalk or a swan or a conch, has an important role to play — that of holding the head at an angle appropriate for a particular emotional situation.

The third item is *shabdam* (song with words), which has four verses, with each giving a dancer the scope to bring out a few interpretations, while introducing short, pure dance sequences between each verse. Thus, the structure of *shabdam* is *abhinaya*-oriented pure dance serving only to provide contrasts to the heavy tract of *abhinaya*. A *shabdam* is usually set in a time-cycle (*tala*) of seven beats called *misra chapu*. To understand the working of elaboration, let us consider the first verse which says, "At the time when lotus-eyed women were bathing, you hid their clothes on a tree, was it proper?" Proceeding from a purely verbal interpretation, a dancer can mime the entire scene of *gopis* (milkmaids) walking to the river bank with water-pots, setting them down to gossip while removing their ornaments and clothes before stepping into the river. They indulge in water-sports — bathing, washing their hair, polishing the pots, filling them with water before stepping out, to find their clothes missing. A solo dancer is at liberty to depict several characters to compliment the actual theme. Thus, the dancer could suggest the character of Krishna holding the flute and reaching the scene to find women bathing when he mischievously collects their clothes, climbs a tree, laughing and mocking while playing on the flute to attract their attention. The dancer can again slide into the characterisation of one of the *gopis*, showing dismay and coquetry alternating with threat and feigned anger. The sequence can be brought to a close by the *gopi* folding her hands in total surrender and receiving her clothes back, to repeat the refrain "Is it proper?" It can be seen from this example that each verse presents the dancer with the possibility of creating a panorama of characters and emotions.

Having undergone the process of learning, the twin aspects of pure and narrational dance, the dancer reaches the stage when she is ripe to embark on the long journey of learning. *Varnam*, an item that has been variously called the masterpiece of Bharatanatyam, the apex of the repertoire and the most difficult dance composition, is indeed like a precious gem, well-cut and well-polished, with each of its facets reflecting effulgence and radiance. In mundane terms, a well-danced *varnam* is like a full meal, comprising the six

LEFT
Shuka sandesh: *A heroine listening to the message brought by her pet parrot which was sent to the hero with a plea of love*
-Sonal Mansingh

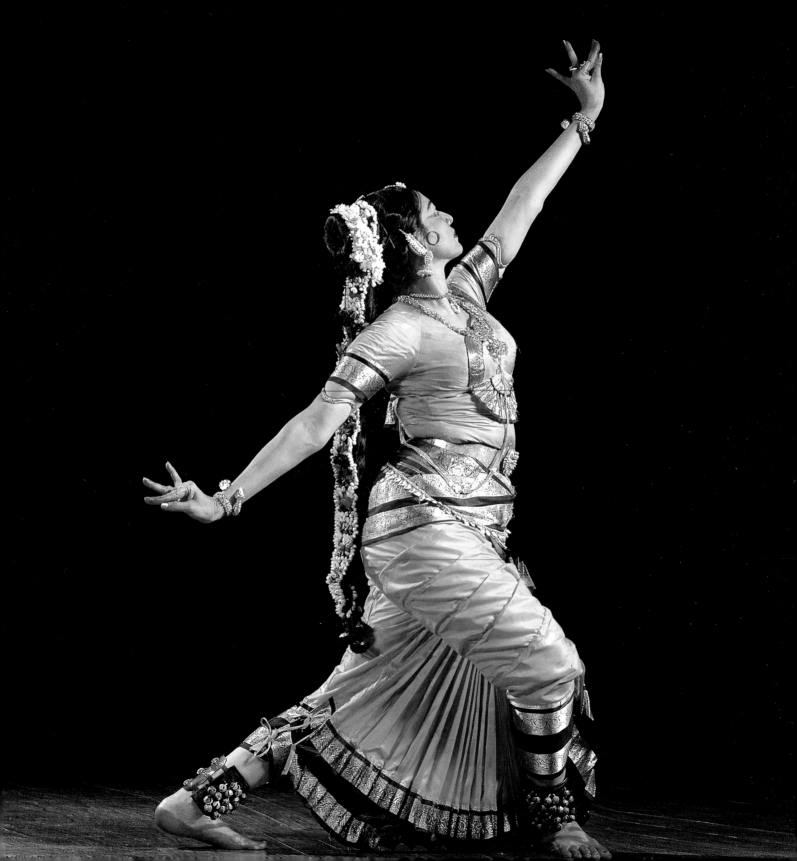

tastes so essential to achieve complete satisfaction. The *shat rasa* or six tastes are:

1. *Katu* - pungent, acrid e.g. hot, chilli
2. *Amla* - sour, acid e.g. vinegar, lemon
3. *Madhur* - honeyed, sweet e.g. sugarcane
4. *Lavan* - saline e.g. salt
5. *Tikta* - bitter e.g. *pichumarda*
6. *Kashaya* - astringent e.g. betel-nut

Varnam is poetry in dance — the kind of poetry which embraces eternal values. The traditional structure of a *varnam* comprises two parts — the first consisting of four verses, each preceded by glittering *jatis* which are especially choreographed to display cross rhythms and dazzling footwork; the second part consists of four or more verses which are preceded by the actual notations of the verse line and are danced at a slightly faster tempo than the first half. Bridging the two parts is a portion called *muktaya*, which sums up the first and hints at the second. From the dance point of view, *varnam* offers a challenge to the dancer, luring her into revealing her powers of interpretation and expression. From the point of view of music too, *varnam* makes demands that the vocalist matches to the cadences of music as per the variegated interpretations of the dance. The vocalist is expected to have a strong sense of rhythm to be able to maintain the *tala* (rhythmic cycle), while the dancer indulges in cross rhythms. A good vocalist can turn a *varnam* into a musical treat, filling it with all the graces of a concert of classical music (*cutcheri*).

The text of a *varnam* usually comes from classical literature and reflects the emotional and philosophical richness. The source material is from the time-honoured epics, *puranas* and the works of saints and poets. A working knowledge of Sanskrit, Tamil, Telugu, and Kannada is deemed essential

The *ragas,* to which the *varnams* are traditionally set, enhance the majestic architecture of the dance. Usually only *ghana* (serious, heavy) *ragas* are used,

LEFT
Widely stretched arms complete the geometry and compliment the leg positions while looking upward at the taut hand-gesture of kataka-mukha *- Yamini Krishnamurthy*

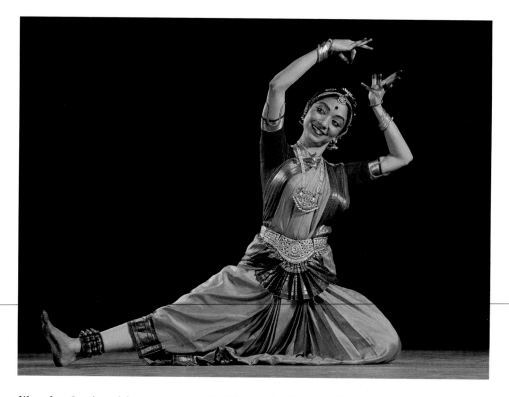

like the Sankarabharanam, Todi, Bhairavi, Kambodhi or Kamas. These are *ragas* which lend themselves to elaborate delineation, giving full scope to an accomplished vocalist to exploit the subtleties while matching the nuances of *abhinaya*. The *varnam* depicts a situation where the *nayika* (heroine) expresses her love for the hero who is either a king or a presiding deity of a temple. This situation calls for a total involvement of the dancer in the role of a *nayika* — now amorous and coquettish, pleading and yearning for his love, more often than not taking her *sakhi* (friend) into confidence. Sometimes a *varnam* is written as a companion's plea to the beloved on behalf of the *nayika*. In both cases the elaboration paints pictures of a soft breeze, moonlit night, flowers in bloom, bees humming and cuckoos calling; in short, all the ingredients supposedly required for creating an atmosphere of desire for love. It depends on the ingenuity of the dancer to breathe new interpretations in the tradition-weary *sanchari bhavas* (transient moods).

Taking *sringara* (love) as the main theme has a distinct advantage. Love in its wake brings in myriad reflections of the *nava rasas* (nine basic moods) and their *sthayibhava, vyabhicharibhava, vibhava* and *anubhava*, as if taking a bird's eye-view of the life around. *Sthayibhava* is the basic and persistent mental state like clear sky. *Vyabhicharibhavas* are the transient emotions like floating clouds. *Vibhavas* mean those circumstances and situations which give rise to and determine the basic mood. *Anubhavas* follow the play of all the above, therefore showing consequent physical activity. Another point that is noteworthy is the parallel meaning, which runs through like a thread holding a necklace. A *varnam* and for that matter most songs danced in India offer the opportunity to be interpreted in two ways — subjective and objective and at two levels — human and divine. It is this constant play between mundane and supra-mundane occurrences in everyday life that is transferred to superhuman beings, endowing the mundane with deeper significance and beauty, while creating an aura of elusive reality. A true devotee of this art travels constantly from one level to another, fusing everyday reality with cosmic dimensions through artistic stylisation and giving the dance a devotional ardour and disciplined abandon.

Hereafter comes the *tillana,* which occurs at the end of the recital. *Tillana* is a pure dance extravaganza exhibiting the exciting possibilities of rhythm-bound vagaries. The *raga* chosen is usually of a lighter and lilting variety as only rhythmic syllables are chanted repeatedly, which do not call for any great musical virtuosity. But the simple arrangement of the music helps enhance the intricate dance structure. The concluding cadences of a *tillana* draw arc-like movements, crisscrossing the stage and bringing a Bharatanatyam recital to an end with rapid-fire dance movements.

Gradually the dancer is introduced to the richness contained in items known as *padams, javali, slokas* and *kirtanams.* These belong to the

PAGE 36
Possibilities of group-work to explore a different dimension of space and time - Chandralekha Dance Company

PAGE 37
The dancer - Chandralekha

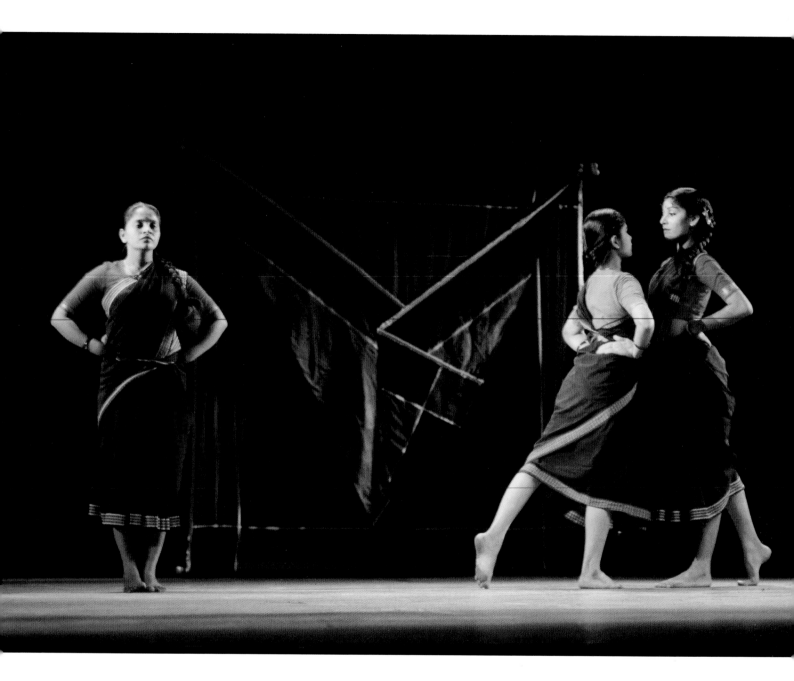

time-honoured secular as well as sacred poetry of poets like Kshetrayya, Tyagaraja, Deekshitar, Shyama Shastri, Swati Thirunal, Dharamapuri Subrayya and some contemporaray names like Papanasam Sivan, Gopala Krishna Bharati, Vasudevacharya, Leelashuka and Ponnah Pillai. *Padams* are songs in Telugu, Tamil, Kannada and Malayalam. *Slokas* are always in Sanskrit. *Javalis* are written in all four southern languages whereas *kirtanams* have been composed mainly in Sanskrit. The *padams* can be of various kinds — extolling the erotic, secular or devotional aspects of love and addressed to a god, a king, or a *nayak* (common man). Most of the *padams* depict a *parakiya nayika* (a woman who is married to another man) yet expresses her love for the hero of the song, be it a nameless man or called by the names of gods like Krishna, Kartikeya or Shiva. This situation calls for careful and deft handling by the dancer who otherwise can slip into overstated eroticism. There are a vast number of songs that speak of innumerable mythological happenings, using rhetoric and epiphany to create

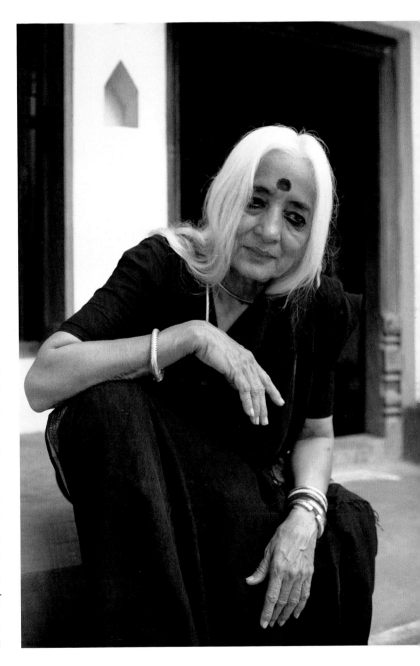

great effect. One such song refers to Vishnu as he is worshipped in the temple of Srirangam in Tamil Nadu where, as Ranganath, he is recumbent on the serpent. The refrain asks: "Why are you asleep, O Lord? Is it because you are exhausted measuring the three worlds as a *vamana* or chasing the golden deer as Rama?"

A wealth of Sanskrit verses known as *slokas* provides the dancer with yet another dimension. Apart from the short verses, the dancer is at liberty to select excerpts from the Sanskrit texts, from epics like the *Ramayana* and *Mahabharata*, the plays of Kalidasa, the *Gita Govinda* of Jayadeva, the *Krishna Karnamrita* of Leelashuka and many others. The devotional hymns of philosophers like Adi Sankaracharya also find a place in a mature dancer's repertoire, because translating philosophical concepts into dance offers a challenge. There is no human activity that has not been written about and extolled.

Having taught the prescribed format called *margam* which includes the repertoire from *allaripu* to *tillana*, the guru makes preparations for the formal presentation of the pupil to the dance world. This event is known as *arangetram* or *rangapravesh* — *ranga* meaning 'stage', and *pravesh* is 'entry'. If the assembled critics and connoisseurs judge the student to be worthy of any future as a dancer, she/he can then continue her/his training with the guru. Thereafter, she/he can also appear in stage performances, usually at the discretion of the guru.

The repertoire as danced today is a creation of the Tanjore quartet, the four brothers — Chinayya, Ponayya, Shivanandam and Vadivelu — who were great scholars and musicians. Before that, Bharatanatyam was a matter of performances going on till the early hours of morning, the dancer haphazardly picking up a few items here and there with long intervals for refreshments and possibly, a snooze. Solo dancing in the temple and in the court was known as Sadir, until early 20th century, when it was christened Bharatanatyam.

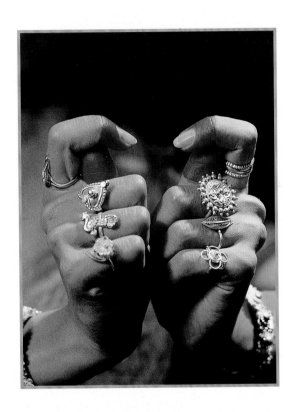

Odissi

PAGE 39
'A pair of birds'

RIGHT
The pleasure of embracing a loved one is clearly visible on the face, posture of the body and band gestures
-Kelucharan Mohapatra

BELOW
A palm-leaf manuscript showing the Trinity of Jagannath, Subhadra and Balabhadra being worshipped in the temple dedicated to Jagannath

The region known as Odra-desh, meaning land of Odra people, formed a strong cultural bond with the adjoining land of Magadh which is part of Bihar state today. Commonality in practice of performing arts merited mention of the dance style as Odramagadhi in the treatise called *Natya Shastra*. Odra-desh was known as Kalinga at the time of Emperor Ashok who fought the infamous Kalinga war in which millions were slaughtered and subsequently made many more grievously wounded and taken captive. Ironically Ashok realised the futility of such bloody excesses and turned to Buddhism for solace. Thus the gallery of sculpted stone caves in Khandagiri hills near Bhubaneswar in Orissa shows King Kharavela and his queen seated on the throne with the royal umbrella held aloft at the back, while enjoying dance and music. Performed by one or more dancers in separate frames, dancers are accompanied by four musicians playing on drums, flute, cymbals and a stringed instrument akin to the *rabab*.

These caves date to 1st century BC. Interestingly the dancers sport a hair-sytle seen in early Gupta and Kushan-period sculptures. Two thick

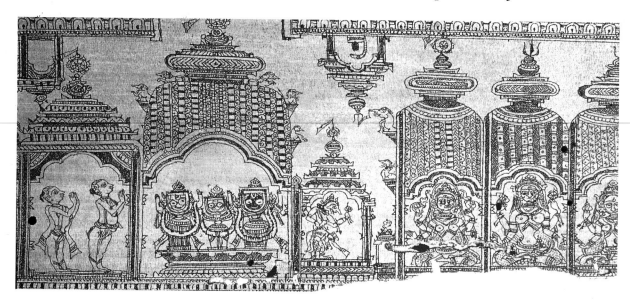

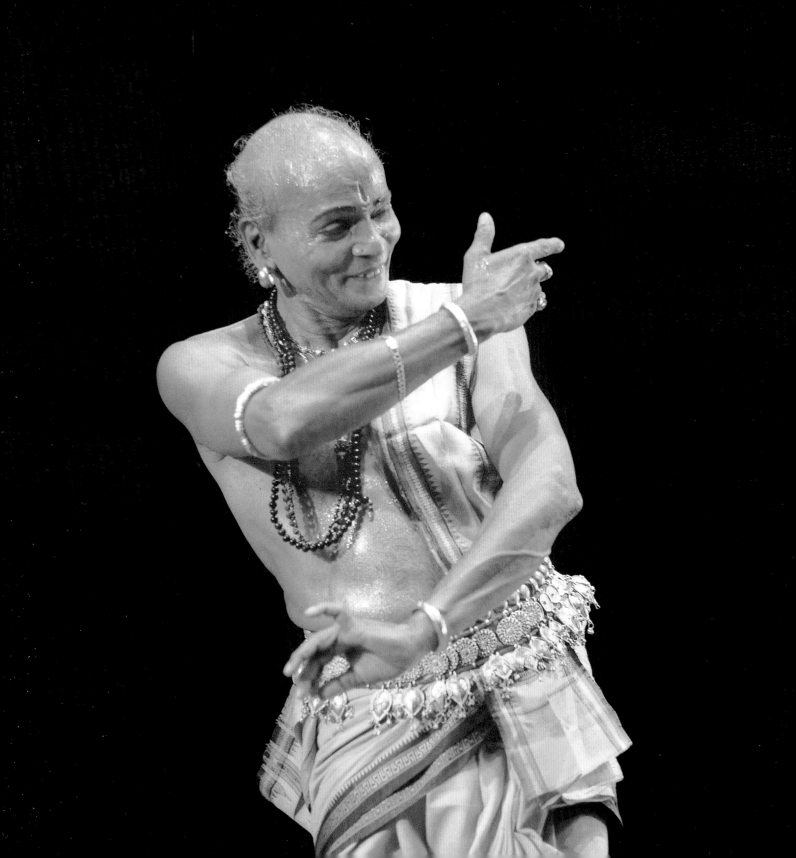

plaits hang over their shoulders reaching almost up to the navel and a huge pendant ornament is fixed at the forehead from where hair is parted. The dancers are tall and well-built with bare, full breasts, slim waists and wearing *ped*, a striped cloth wrap, around the lower waist and legs in the style of a *sarong* or *lungi*. Their bangles and ankle ornaments are thick and rather unembellished. Such a representation of dance in a performance is rare to find in stone from such an early period. Besides serving as a proof of dance as an art performance in royal courts, there are enough depictions of dance for the populace. The style of dressing and costumes of dancers show them as having come from far off lands.

Odra-desh, Kalinga and then Utkal merged into the political identity of Orissa state from where the dance style derives its name, Orissi or Odissi. Down the centuries dance continued to flourish with royal patronage and popular support so that when temple-building activity started, dancing became an integral part of the temple rituals. Following the ruler's preferred religion, the temples had Shiva, Vishnu, *Surya* (Sun), Devi and their various manifestations as presiding deities.

The Parasurameshwar temple of 6th century AD has some interesting sculptures of Shiva as Lakulisa, in strong dance postures. In a unique concept of worship, the temples sported a plethora of sculptures on the outer walls showing not only geometrical patterns, tresses, flowers, birds and animals, stories from the well known texts like the *Ramayana, Mahabharata* and *Bhagawad*, but also vivid figures of female dancers in postures described in the *Natya Shastra*. They played on musical instruments, held a mirror to look at their own beauty, stood langurously awaiting a lover or just lazing under a tree, held a parrot or warded off a monkey pulling at clothes, squeezed out water from long, washed hair, drops from which fall into the eagerly open beak of a swan, played with a ball or combed thick hair into an elaborate hairdo, applying *kajal* (kohl) to their fish-shaped eyes or a *tilak* on the forehead. Women were depicted as a dancer, a lover, a musician, a

RIGHT
The tribhangi *posture forms one of the two basic stances of Odissi dance vocabulary. Three flexions at the neck, hip and knee are worked into various compositions, both of pure dance,* nritta *or expressive dance,* nritya *and* abhinaya
-Sonal Mansingh

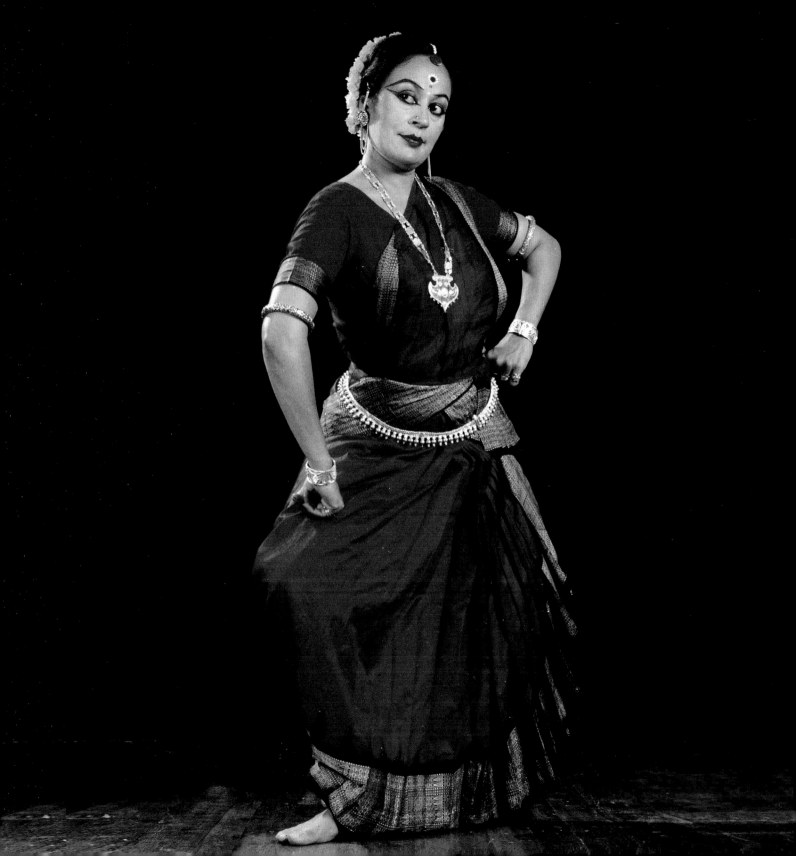

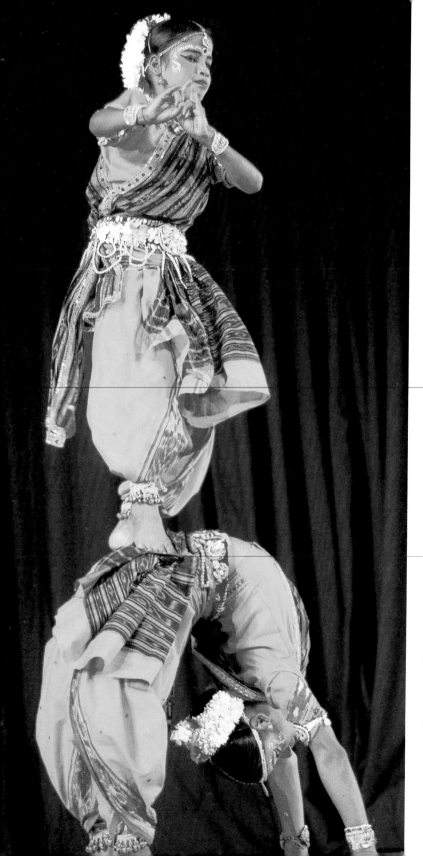

mother, a traveller, a teacher, a goddess, as if life was one huge temple in which everything around the human being was reconciled and beautified.

As if to counterbalance the galaxy of female sculptures, many temples show images of a dancing Shiva in various forms pertaining to the many Saivite legends. Shiva as the loving husband of Parvati, Shiva riding the Nandi bull, Shiva as Bhairava, Shiva as Tripura Samhara and many more sculptures adorning the temple-walls became books in stone from which iconography of each god and goddess could be learnt. It is very important for an Indian dancer, specially a dancer of Odissi, to know the stories connected with each Divinity and his depiction in stone sculptures or wood panels and in mural paintings for they form the vocabulary of the danced texts peopled with divine and demonic characters, sages and kings, lovers and mendicants. As with Shiva, so with Vishnu in his 10 incarnations or in the deep ocean lying on a serpent–bed with Goddess Lakshmi, his consort, or standing alone with the four arms holding a conch, discus, mace and lotus. Vishnu as Krishna, the naughty blue god with a flute, is usually shown in the *tribhanga*, the three-bend posture, as he plays on the flute, or dances with the women from Vrindavan and Gokul — the pastoral villages on the banks of River Yamuna, or kills the demonic forces appearing in various forms — as a huge crane, an uncontrollable horse, a crazed elephant, an endless python, a wicked sorceress, a gust of terrifying storm, an unquenchable fire or an angry and arrogant Indra sending down torrential rains and storms for seven days and nights, drowning the entire region when Krishna lifted Mount Govardhan to provide shelter to people of Vrindvan. His love for cows and calves, whom he took to graze in the forest, his mischievous pranks, his uncanny ways of pleasing men, women, children, bird and beast alike, his hunger for sweet butter churned by the women of Gokul for which he could break into homes or forcibly take it from the women — all these and more form the basis of the narrative dance

LEFT
Aerobatic feats have been a part of training of young male dancers dressed as girls. They are known as Gotipua

BELOW
Intense devotion can be shown through dance
- Sharmila Biswas

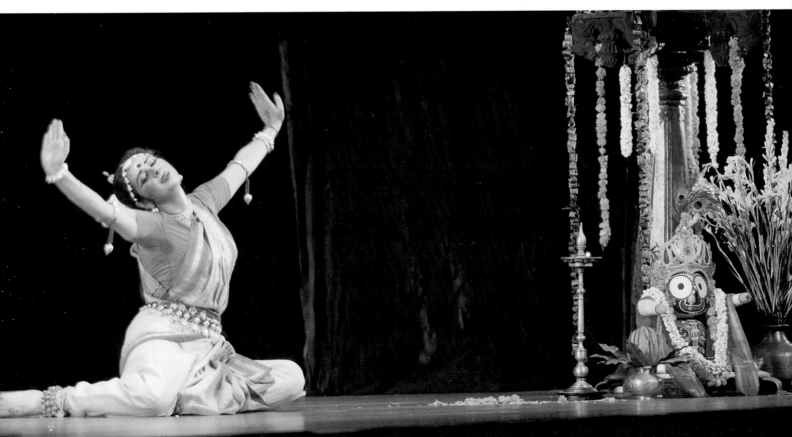

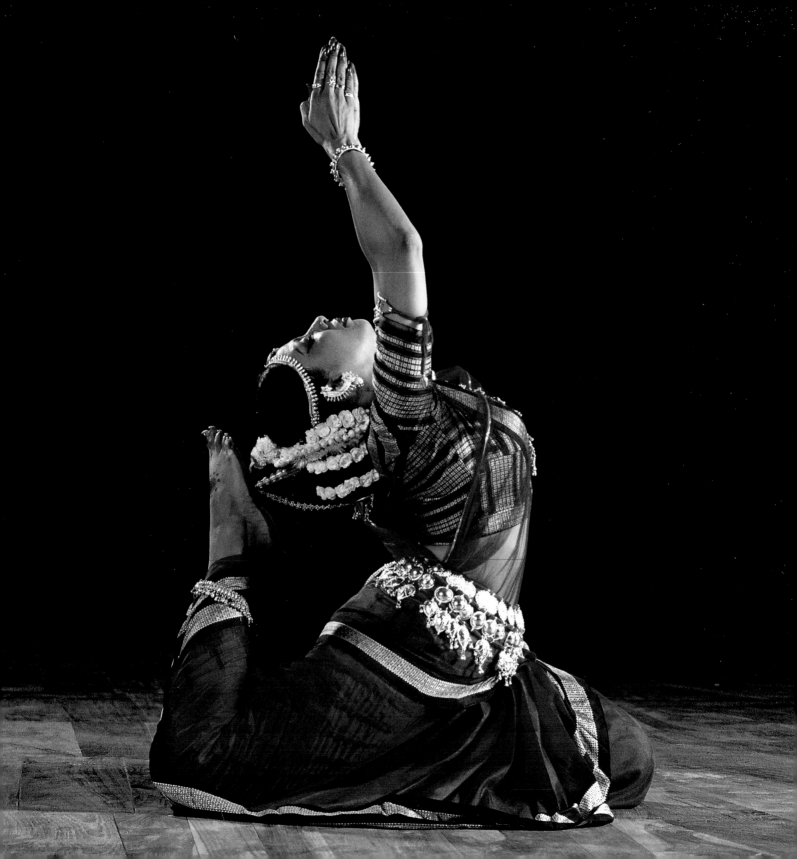

in Odissi. Stories, parables, poems, and plays, both in oral and written traditions, tell us of the great love of Krishna for an older Radha who was the epitome of love, grace, and beauty.

Radha and Krishna have long been a symbol of unconditional love and of transcending all known human barriers that belittle and trivialise love. Among the vast number of literature on the subject, the *Gita Govinda* by poet Jayadev stands out as an all-time great love-poem. He lived in the 12th century and was married to a beautiful dancer, Padmavati. Both were devotees of Jagannath, lord of the universe, whose majestic temple stands at Puri on the south-eastern shores of India. The interchangeability of names, forms and attributes as well as stories of one god with many of his own incarnations and manifestations have confused many, who are unaware of the simple truth at the root of this seemingly confusing multiplicity. The truth is about ourselves and our many faces, moods and forms during one single day, not to speak of a lifetime. Therefore, Vishnu in his eighth incarnation is called Krishna. Both share common attributes of form and intent. Krishna wears a *peetambara*, a yellow garment, which shines like the golden streak of lightning on his blue body and so does Vishnu. For any interested reader, the symbolism of blue as space and yellow as the shimmer of cosmic light would be amply clear. Vishnu is at once dark, black-blue. As Jagannath he represents the unmanifest, that which existed before creation. Here he is accompanied by Shakti, the cosmic energy, that triggers, empowers and galvanises pure matter which is still dark and unknown. She is golden and is called Subhadra. At the touch of energy, vibrations begin and the black and unknown, the pure matter revealing itself in myriad forms. Therefore the manifested form is white and is known as Balabhadra. Thus Vishnu as Jagannath and Vishnu as Krishna are equal to Jagannath. Krishna's life history and the geography of his various peregrinations are recorded in the *Srimad Bhagawad* and the epic *Mahabharata*. The Odissi dancer smoothly sails across these various streams to find the

LEFT
Offering prayers with body and soul
- Protima Bedi

one essence — that divine from which enchants the mind, fills the eyes and enriches the life.

Of similar nature and scope are the other characters of Devi, the great goddess with a million names; Ganesha the elephant-headed god of wisdom; the Sun-god with the lotus symbol and riding a chariot pulled by seven horses (which stands for seven days); and Shiva, who alone does not have any incarnations and yet is always present as this popular verse suggests: "The universe is his body; every sound, vibration, word, music are his speech; the Sun, moon, and stars adorn him as jewels, to such cosmic beatitude, called Shiva, to whom I bow."

To imbibe and translate grand ideas, images and concepts, the dancer has to go through a regimen of exercises and postures while learning different kinds of walks, jumps, leaps and runs typical to the style of Odissi. Although Odissi shares a family resemblance to Bharatanatyam, it is informed by a totally different philosophy of form. By using the upper torso as an independent unit, Odissi makes the torso glide from side to side in a smooth sway. Combined with the frequent use of *tribhanga* (thrice-bent posture) and the gentle, oblique movement of the neck, Odissi can remind a viewer of watching a piece of fine filigree or a creeper gently swaying in a soft breeze. Yet Odissi is not just *lasya*, feminine grace. The *chowka bhangi*, creating a square with the half-seated posture, both knees turned outwards and both hands stretched at shoulder level and then bent outwards from the elbow, can be heavy duty, more so when various leaps, jumps, and stamps to a given rhythmic cycle (*tala*) have to be executed according to a demanding choreography. Most basic dance patterns are learnt both in *chowka* and *tribhanga* postures in fully seated (on toes, knees out) or half seated (on toes, heels or flat feet) or standing in *sama, abhanga* or *tribhanga*.

Odissi found its modern *avatar* in 1959 when a repertory was built by combining elements from the prevalent performing art traditions of Orissa, like Chhau, Sabda-Swara, Patha, Sakhi Naach, Geeti Natya, Ras Lila, etc.

RIGHT
An enchanting glimpse of sheer feminine grace -Sanjukta Panigrahi

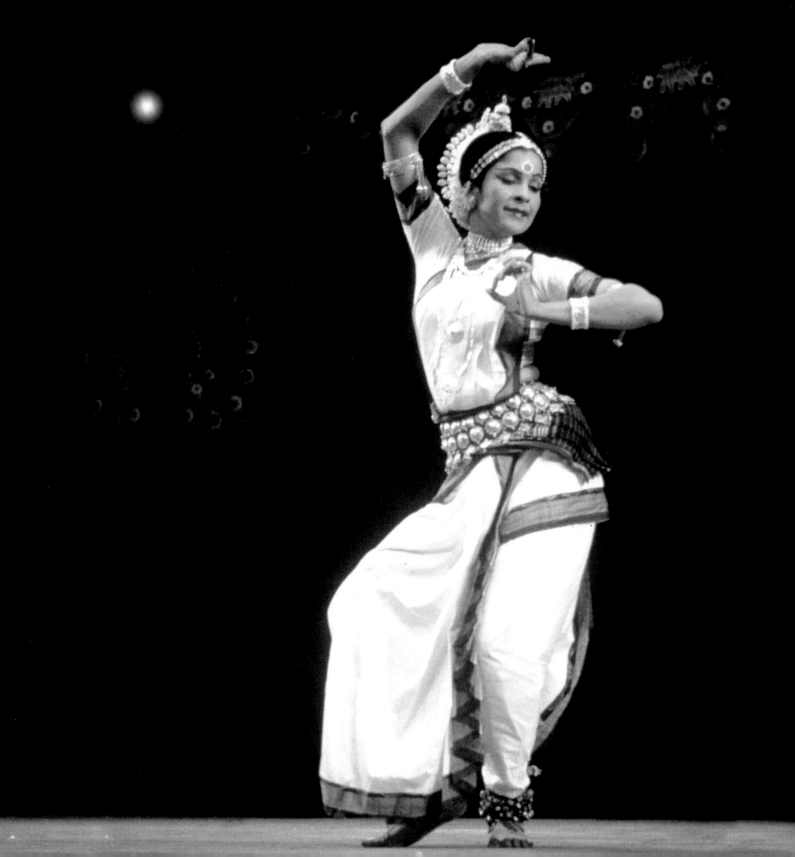

Since then, the repertory includes *mangalacharan* (auspicious beginning, a prayer), *batu* or *sthaayi* (composition showing typical postures of Odissi mostly seen in sculptures), *pallavi* (a music composition in a particular musical mode), *raga* (with a complex rhythmic pattern), *geet, shloka, champu, ashtapadi* (poems as music compositions allowing for detailed treatment of expansive and communicative *abhinaya*) and *natangi* or *mokshya* as the final homage to creation through dance.

Odissi has spread its scope immensely and now boasts of choreographies on every conceivable theme using ancient, medieval and modern poetry. The accompanying music needs special mention as being truly indigenous to Orissa and comprising many *ragas* and *talas* unique to Odissi. The orchestra for the dance usually consists of a vocalist, a *pakhawaj* (percussion instrument), a flute and violin or the *sitar*.

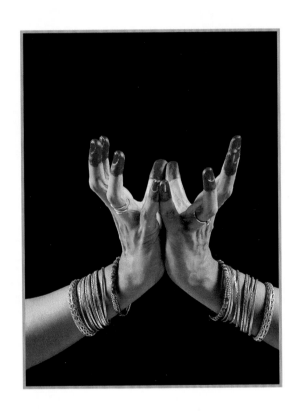

Kathak

PAGE 51
'A lotus'

As the name suggests, Kathak is a by-product of the art of story-telling in ancient India. In Sanskrit, a story is *katha*, therefore story-tellers came to be known as *kathaks*, rather than by the longer word, *kathakar*. Perhaps the city-bred may not be familiar with this typical rural entertainment where the whole village gathers around a man fluently reciting from the well-known epics and legends. As he speaks, his eyes shine, his hands gesticulate, his toes curl, and he sweeps his audience into the world of valour and romance, of gods and goddesses, intrigues and jealousies, battles and victories. Like a conjurer he creates a world peopled by larger than-life characters, now bursting into a song, then in rising excitement breaking into a few graceful steps using his hands to describe the coyness of a Radha or the courage of a fighting Arjuna.

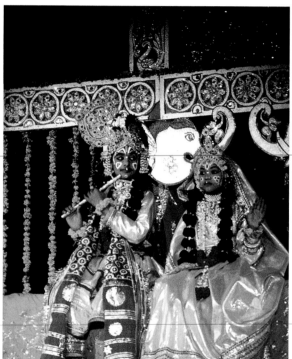

The theatre is the platform under a spreading tree which otherwise serves as a meeting place for village elders in times of peace. The *kathaks* are artists well-versed in lore and human psychology. The ease with which they generate responses and reactions is an index of the affinity between an art which is verbal-cum-visual and the sensibilities of a basically innocent yet sensitive people.

It seems that temple-building activity in the north encouraged the parallel activities of music and dance which, as in other parts of India, were used as vehicles of worship. *Sevadars* were the counterparts of the *kathaks* in the temples; they played on the *pakhawaj* and sang in front of the lord. This activity produced the great system of music now known as Dhrupad. In time, the music was accompanied by simple movements, of ritual offering and recounting the glory of god, which created a distinct style of performance imbued with

ABOVE
Radha and Krishna, the Divine lovers. Vrindavan and Mathura in North India echo with songs and recounting of deeds and life of Krishna is common practice - Dancers from Vrindavan

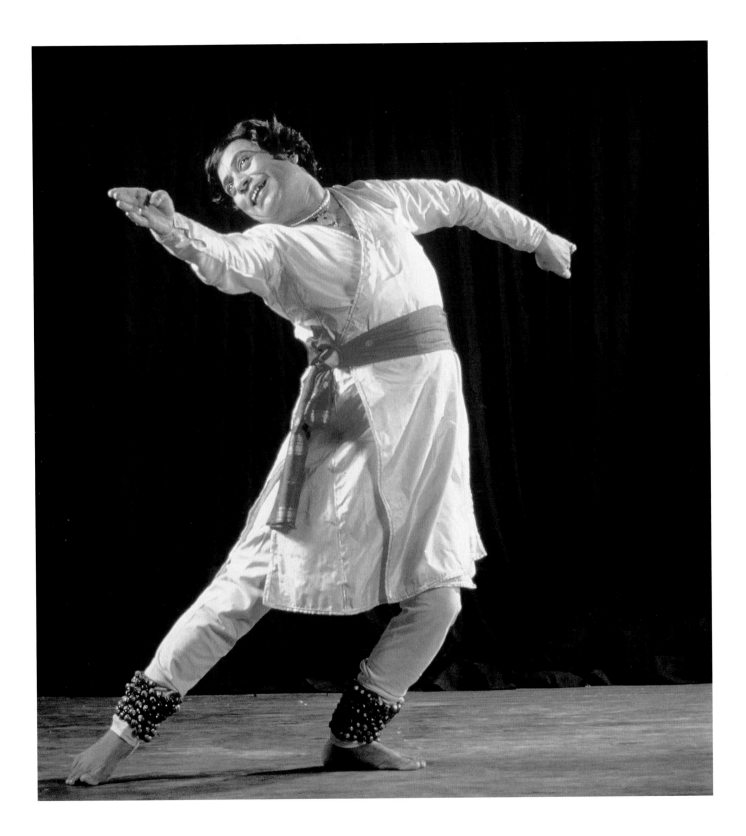

beatified devotion. As a consequence of the ravages wrought by the successive waves of invaders, there is little evidence left of the exact nature of the kind of temple dance that existed during the centuries up to the 16th century AD.

Relief from the monotony of constant wars and destruction came in the form of a resurgence of sentiments and devotion in the poems of such mystics as Kabir, Surdas, Mira, Tulsidas, Raskhan, Behari, Vidyapati and Chandidas among others. The beauty of their language and inner vision encouraged people at large to weave them into their daily duties and build an edifice of dance and music which came to be called Ras Lila.

Vraja *bhumi*, the land where Krishna played as a child and grew to manhood, has special significance in Kathak. The area around Mathura and Vrindavan is considered so sacred that even the trees, creepers, animals and birds, not to mention the dust of this area, are worshipped. The *Dasham Skandha* of the *Bhagawad Purana* comes alive through the *kathak* who revels in the dance of the milkmaids, speaks of Krishna as a beautiful boy and extols the virtue of love and devotion through total surrender in love.

The Ras Lila is a circular dance performed by men and women swaying gracefully to the beats of the *mridang* and the *pakhawaj*, to the melody of the *veena* and flute played by none other than Krishna himself. The circular dance goes on until mood and movement emerge from every limb, and the milkmaids and the multi-formed Krishna become one. It is this Ras Lila which is symbolic of the eternal play between the soul and god that has been the focal point of Kathak in earlier times.

Historically in the reign of Nawab Wajid Ali Shah of Oudh (19th century AD) Kathak gained in prominence and spread. Contrary to the strict Islamic tradition, the Nawab provided a shining example of tolerance, while even dressing as Krishna and dancing to the songs on Krishna, written by himself, in the company of court dancers dressed as milkmaids. The Lucknow School of Kathak was thus established with the involvement of the royal

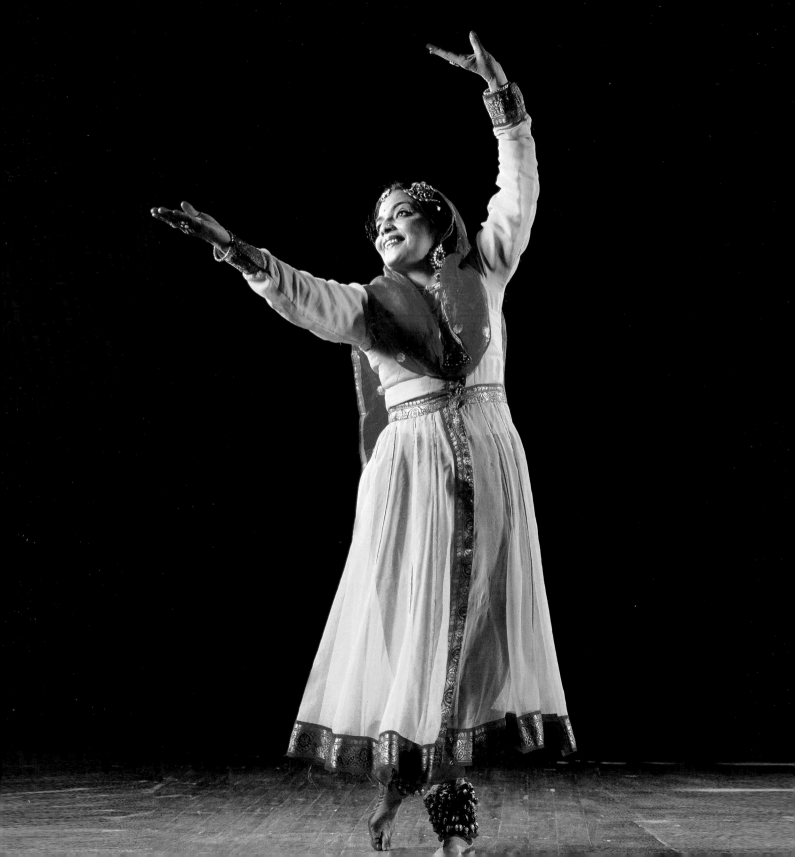

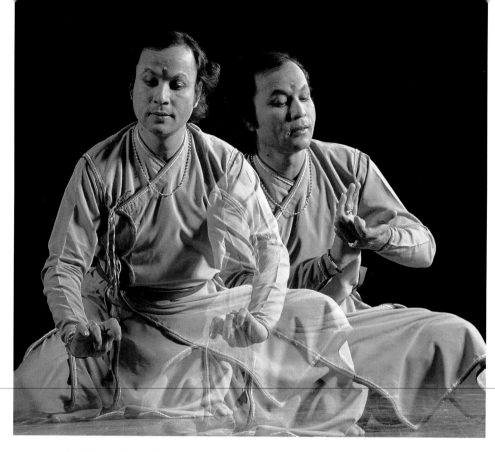

patron. He brought Thakur Prasad, whose two sons, Binda Din and Kalka Prasad, succeeded him at the court. Kalka Prasad's forte was his mastery of rhythm, whereas Binda Din was a composer of no mean merit, excelling specially in *thumris, dadras,* and *ghazals.* Thus, the Lucknow *gharana* of Kathak acquired its pleasing synthesis of rhythm and grace.

Apart from the Lucknow *gharana*, there are two distinct schools, namely, the Jaipur and Benaras. Jai Lal and Sunder Prasad left an indelible stamp on the rhythmic aspect of Kathak. The Benaras *gharana* came into prominence with Sukhdev Maharaj.

The orchestra reveals the predominance of percussion instruments. The *pakhawaj, tabla*, the *nakra*, and the *manjira* provide the exciting possibilities of how rhythm alone can raise dance to unimaginable heights. The other members of the orchestra are usually a vocalist and a *sarangi* player. The recital proper begins with an invocation to Ganesha as is traditional among other dance styles also. This may be a simple *shloka* or song in Hindustani or Sanskrit, danced with simple gestures, without indulging in complex pure dance patterns. After the obeisance to god comes the salutation to the audience with an *aamad* (entry) and *salaami*. The dancer establishes the atmosphere with slow and graceful movements signifying salutation, either as a *pranam* in the Hindu way, or as a *salaam* in the Islamic way. The *aamad* is the act of entering the stage formally, after which follows the *thaat* — a static pose showing Krishna as the *nata-nagar*. The right hand is extended vertically above the head, signifying the peacock feather, the insignia of Krishna. The left arm is extended horizontally to the left, signifying his embracing of Radha, his beloved. The subtle movements of the wrist, the amorous glances of the eyes, the graceful horizontal gliding of the neck, the tremulous fluttering of the fingers and eyebrows help to invoke an atmosphere reminiscent of the days when emperors and courtiers sat around, in their glittering jewels and brocades, casting admiring glances at

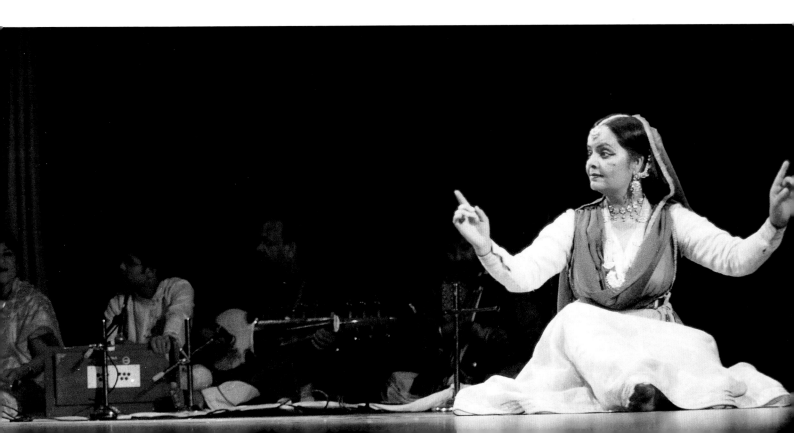

the *houri* — the heavenly dancer who is the reward for virtuous followers of Islam.

Hereafter the dancer is ready to take up the introductory elements, like the *gat*. This word comes from the Sanskrit root *gam-gachhati*, meaning 'to go', 'to move', 'to cover space'. Thus the *gat* is a phrase that denotes locomotion, and is representative of themes and characters easily recognisable by the way the dancer moves forward, takes a *palta* (changing direction), slides from one character to another, glides in to *gat-nikas* (steps rhythmically backwards) characterising the essential features of the item.

In the episode of Kailya-*damana* (victory over Kaliya, the cobra king) the dancer would perhaps begin the *gat-bhava* by showing Krishna in his characteristic pose of playing the flute. River Yamuna is then shown with rippling hand movements. The cows are shown grazing and other cowherds playing around. The dancer shows with her hand gestures a cow drinking water and falling dead. The eyes move rapidly in horror to show a similar fate befalling all the characters except Krishna, who has climbed a tree to survey the river before jumping into the river. The dancer then mimes the ensuing battle between Krishna and the poisonous snake, Kaliya. After a few symbolic postures and steps, where the accompanying music also reaches a crescendo, Krishna is shown dancing triumphantly on the hood of the cobra. The *gat-nikas* holds the posture of triumphant Krishna while treading lightly, covering the stage backwards and arriving at the *sam* (the defining beat of a time-cycle) perfectly on time.

All along the *sarangi* player plays a melodious composition set to a particular time-cycle which is called *lehar*. It accompanies this segment of the recital where it fulfils the need of the dancer to ensure alternate and quick-change portrayals. The time is now ripe for a leisurely delineation of *bhava* (moods) that would cover such popular types of musical compositions like *dadra*, *thumri*, *ghazal* and *bhajan*. The tempo of the recital at this stage is slow enough to allow detailed rendering.

RIGHT
A posture of teasing majesty
- Sitara Devi

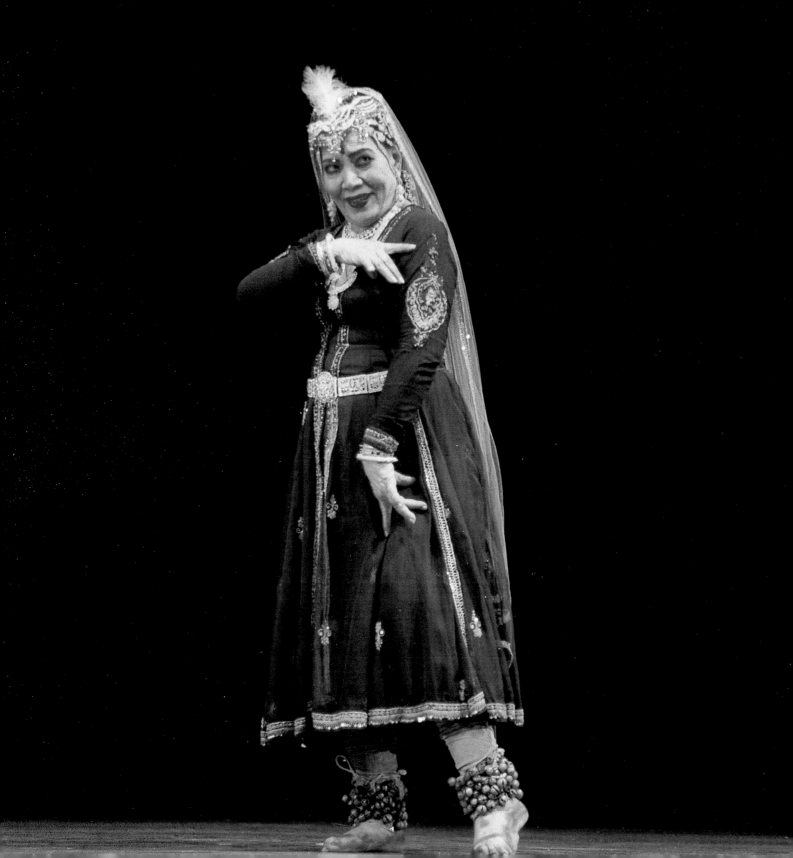

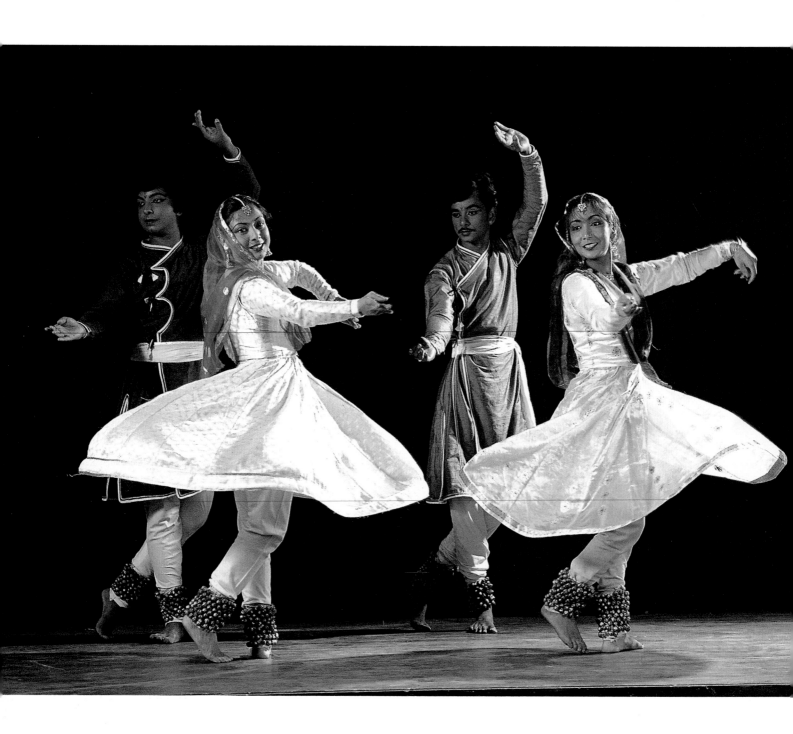

Kathak does not use a number of hand gestures, as do Bharatanatyam and Odissi. It uses, rather, the entire body to convey the import of the song.

Hereafter the dancer tackles passages of pure dance with unrestrained gusto, entering into frequent bouts with the percussionists. Beginning with *tukras*, which are pieces of pure dance set to complex rhythmic permutations within the given time-cycle, the dance progresses apace with the introduction of *parans* and *paramelus*. Whereas the *tukras* are accompanied by the *tabla* (a two-piece percussion instrument), the *paramelus* interweave an intricate pattern of rhythms played on one or on all the percussion instruments together. Alternately the unique syllables of the *tabla, pakhawaj*, the *nakra* (percussion drums of different sizes and tones) are combined in one rhythmic passage, thus creating a *paramelu* (*para* meaning 'different', *melu* meaning 'union'). As can be imagined, these pieces offer a great variety and scope to the dancer and the percussionists. Since these are danced at great speed, an absolute understanding of the *talas* (time-cycles) and their implications are essential. A perfect command over the limbs and their velocity while in fast action is another requirement also — a body that is perfectly balanced even at the end of a demanding series of pirouettes. All this time the *lehar* plays unerringly at a steady pace on the *sarangi*, providing anchor to the fast-moving dancer.

The dancer may do this at the end of just a couple of rounds of the time-cycle or go on weaving complex rhythmic patterns for several more rounds until her mental calculations propel her towards the vortex. If she calculates correctly, she would land on the *sam* as an arrow hits the bull's eye. If her mind wavers, she could land on a wrong beat, much to her embarrassment and of the orchestra, and the audience. But when the dancer arrives at the *sam* correctly, an audible sigh runs through the audience. The concept of *vishranti* (repose) is all-important and equally applicable to all performing arts in India because the natural law of physical dynamics dictates that there be an ebb after the tide, i.e. a point of stillness.

LEFT
Pandit Birju Maharaj's disciples presenting Kathak dance

Like the flow of a river that quickens near the ocean, the tempo of the programme increases at every stage, particularly now with the eddying and swirling of the dance called *tatkar*. These are the climatic moments with the dancer manipulating the pace of footwork, weaving in and out of the complexities, luring the drummer on to false trails, engaging him in a quick-silver bout of extempore responses, pitting her wits against his in keeping up the cadences of variegated footwork, controlling the sound of ankle-bells of which 150 are worn on the left foot and 150 on the right. A hush invariably falls over the audience as the dancer controls the sound of ankle-bells, bringing it to an ever-decreasing level and finally controlling the muscles and nerves to an extent that only one tinkling bell is heard. In a trifle, the sound increases gradually to its original pitch and joins the drummer in a vigorous display of final frenzy. The recital is brought to a close in the manner of a swashbuckling Samurai and with a triumphant look, the dancer makes her exit.

Two kinds of costumes have gained currency among female Kathak dancers. One is the hip to ankle-long, full-pleated skirt which is usually in bright colours worked over with gold or silver threads. A short blouse of matching material and colour adorns the torso and a long gossamer scarf is tucked in at one end at the waist in the style of Hindu women of North India. The ornaments are usually based on old designs and studded with precious or semi-precious stones. The other costume represents Islamic influence. A tight pyjama, usually of a bright and contrasting colour, is worn under a high-necked diaphanous dress, called the *angharkha* in which the bodice is tight, outlining the contours, while the lower half swings out in full gathers. *Kathak* dancers can draw freely upon the vast store-house of Hindi and Urdu literature as also the works of poets who wrote in regional versions of Hindi like Braj, Awadhi, Maithili, and Hindustani.

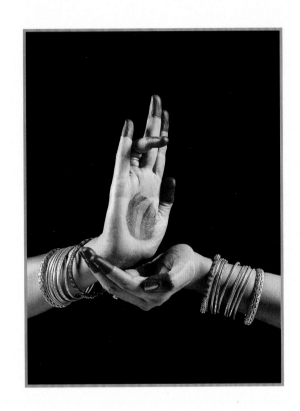

Kathakali

Dusk is falling. A soft breeze blows with the ripened paddy swaying in the entire field at its will. Tall palms rustle, the red earth tinging the landscape like a ruby set amidst an emerald-green verdure. The rumble grows louder. People hurry out of their homes and fields to surround the drummers who are announcing the staging of a Kathakali play that night. There is time to have the evening meal, change clothes, prepare the children for the evening and still find a vantage seat in the area surrounding the arena, which will be used as a stage.

Night has fallen. Two enormous brass lamps, lit with wicks soaked in coconut oil, throw long shadows. The children play, the women gossip, men smoke *bidis* or chew betelnut, talk of this and that when, again, the drum-beats engage their attention. The vanguard consists of percussionists, one playing on the *chenda*, barrel-shaped vertical drum, emitting ear-splitting, blood-curdling sounds; another playing on the *maddalam*, the horizontal drum. Then comes another beating the basic time-cycle on a pair of large cymbals. This is the prologue to the play proper which will go on for the entire night. With the drums and cymbals reaching a crescendo, a portable cloth curtain is brought in, and held by two men dressed like musicians in the typical Kerala fashion — bare-bodied with a *mundu*, a single piece of fine cotton wrapped around the waist. This curtain is the beginning of the *lila*, the play that is to unfold.

The curtain has a symbolic significance — it befogs our vision and needs to be removed if reality has to be glimpsed. The main character of the first scene of a particular play also walks in with the curtain and begins behind it his ritualistic worship of the stage and instruments and offers salutations to the gods. All the while the music carries on, with the curtain-bearers nonchalantly holding the tassels' ends. Suddenly a hand, with long silver-tipped nails appears, and the fingers curl and uncurl, now grabbing the curtain, now releasing it. The hand disappears and a blood-curdling shriek is heard. A magnificent, multi-tiered crown comes into view, casting

PAGE 63
'The lamp'

RIGHT
Kalamandalam
Krishna Nair

a spell over the now agitated and eager audience. The crown sways, two hands grab the edge of the screen, release it violently, making the curtain-bearers almost swerve and fall. The crown disappears from view. High-pitched drumming follows the apparently energetic back-screen dancing, bringing it to a point where the eyes, like burning coals, heavily outlined by kohl, mesmerise the audience. The powerful glance shifts jerkily in all directions, taking in as if every single onlooker, challenging, mocking, inviting. Again, the eyes with the crown disappear. Thus it goes on. For a time the character plays hide and seek, revealing and yet not revealing and, aided by constant drumming, creating almost unbearable tension until, with a demonic shriek and a furious leap, the curtain is dropped to show the full glory of this larger-than-life character. Audible gasps receive this apparition from another world — a world of gods and demons, of saintly beings and sinners, of the absolute belief that good triumphs over evil. A performance of Kathakali now begins.

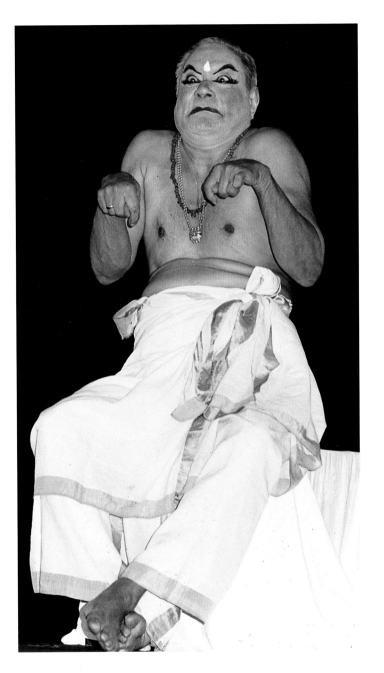

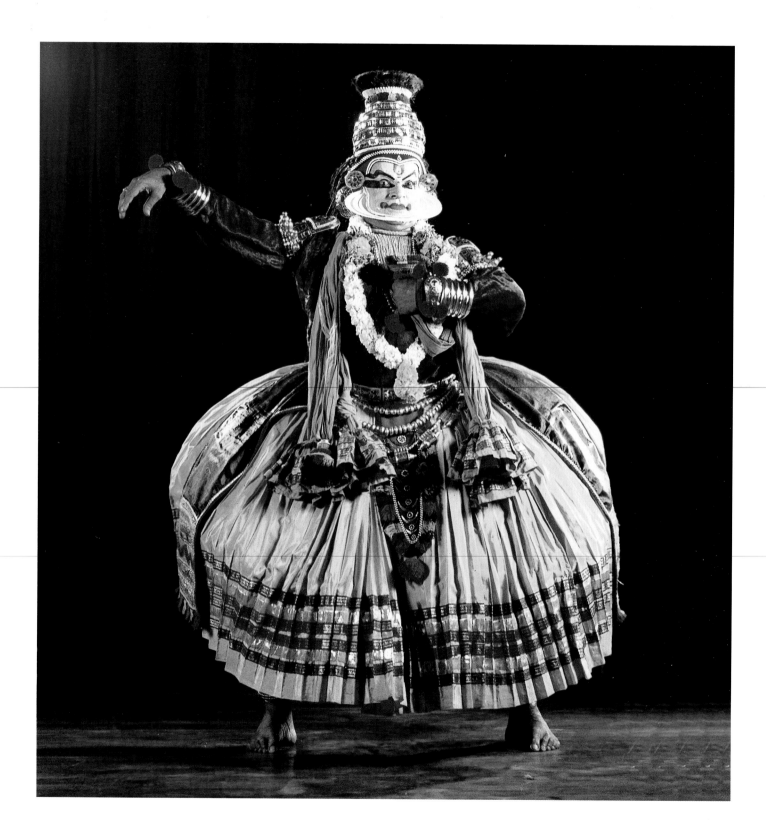

performed the story of Rama equally proficiently. The present form of Kathakali largely derives from these two immediate predecessors. The use of drums and vocal singing was introduced in Krishnanattam because the stories had to be recited and enunciated clearly. In Ramanattam, the use of *chenda*, the barrel-shaped vertical drum, added volume and tonal variations which enriched the scope of characterisation. Vocal singing attained more prominence with the two singers rushing to match the long duration of the eight-night performance. The masks gave way to elaborate make-up and headgear clearly defined into different types. The legend has it that the Raja of Kottayam saw Lord Vishnu emerging from the Milky Ocean in a dream. Just as his vision took in the details of the Lord's beauty, magnificence and attributes, the dream ended, alas, leaving behind the memory of the billowing waves after which he fashioned the billowing skirts of his dancers. Such a legend must be given credence to account for the unexpected sight of many yards of cloth whirling around. Continued royal patronage fed the channels, enriching the twin streams and making it almost a privileged duty to

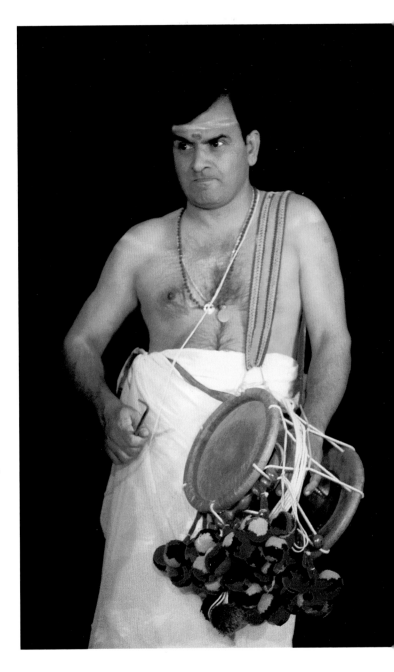

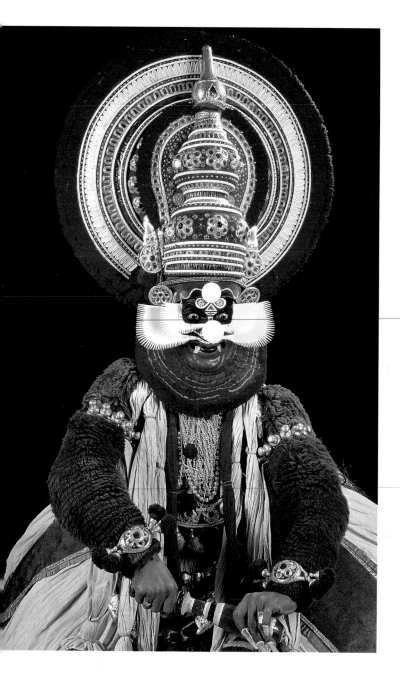

patronise, propagate and present these dance-dramas. Krishnanattam in particular, by being danced in the temple at Guruvayur, led the way to the later exposure of Kathakali to all peoples, irrespective of their caste and religion.

The author of the first four dance-dramas written specially for enactment was the scholarly Raja of Kottayam. The themes chosen were naturally from the *Mahabharata*. Subsequently the Mahahraja of Tranvancore and Vidvan Koyil Thampuran enriched the repertoire. In contemporary times, two names stand out for their contribution to the literary richness. They are Unnayi Warrier and Irayimman Thampi. It is believed there are around 150 works written for Kathakali out of which about 100 are published for ready reference. Out of these, about 40 form the repertoire of Kathakali today. But according to experts only 20 of these are regular features. Most of the themes for these dance-dramas are derived from *Devi Bhagavatham*, the *Mahabharata*, the *Ramayana* and the *Bhagawad Purana*. Therefore the themes are well known, easily understood and capable of being appreciated by connoisseurs as well as the commoner.

Highly-stylised vocabulary of hand-gestures and eye movements characterise this dance-theatre. Also specialised make-up in vivid colours and designs on the face distinguish each character. A god or a hero would have green background as the basic colour on the face while a royal character with violent temperament would have red. The red could be used even for anti-gods, for kings like Ravana who challenged the good and just Prince Rama to battle. Black paint as background colour on face is used for those who live in forests, on mountains or are different from the generally accepted civilised society. Yellow make-up is used for females as well as for mendicants, sages and saintly characters.

To savour the multi-layered subtleties of Kathakali, indeed of any of the classical dance forms of India, the audience is expected to be equally

LEFT
A ferocious and awesome character who appears to strike terror in the hearts of the audience with the huge crown, exaggerated whiskers and red beard - Sadanam Balakrishnan

BELOW
Scene from a dance-drama - Dancers from International Centre for Kathakali

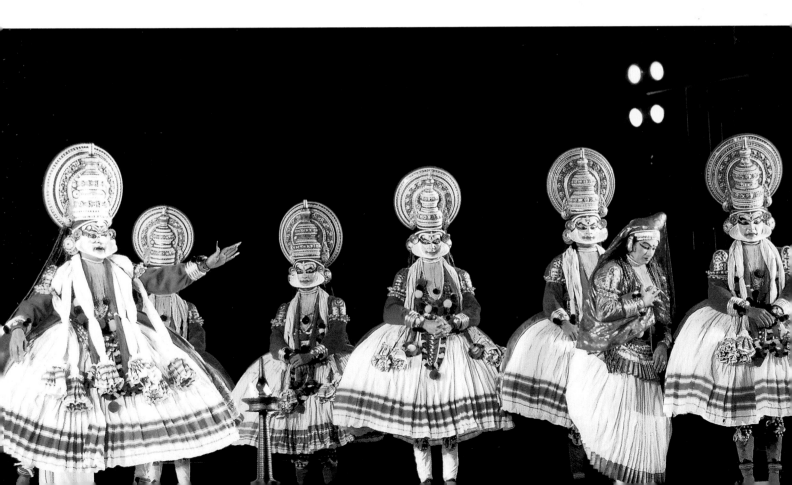

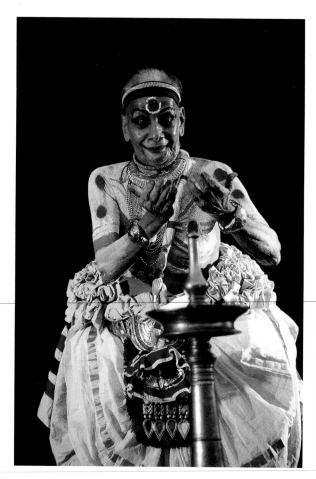
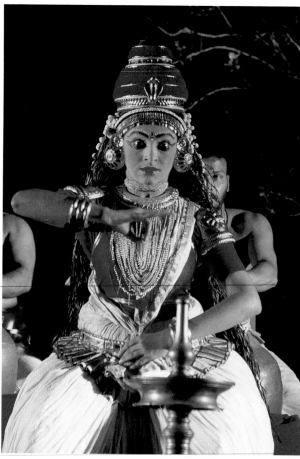

ABOVE
The ancient Sanskrit theatre, Kudiyattam - Amanoor Madhav Chakiar

receptive and knowledgeable. The terms often used for such an informed viewer is *rasika* who is "the lover of the beautiful. Also, it could be anyone who has a healthy sense of humour and wit, anyone who enjoys the pleasures of life, anyone who can create an atmosphere of cheer and happiness around him" (quoted from K. Bharatha Iyer).

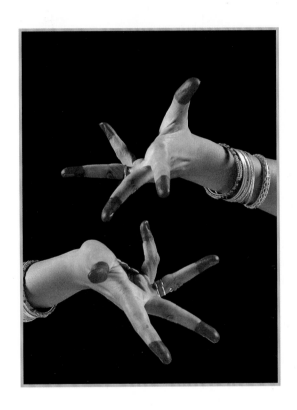

Manipuri

Manipur is a compound of two words in Sanskrit — *mani* means 'jewel' and *pur* mean 'land' or 'city'. Indeed the verdant foliage of the valleys of Manipur with hundreds of varieties of orchids, mushrooms, flowers, shrubs, and other such bounties of Nature justify the name given to this land bordering Myanmar on the east and Bangladesh on the west. Manipur nestles in the far corner of the north-eastern states in India. The epic *Mahabharata* mentions Manipur in the context of the valiant hero Arjuna's incognito visit and his subsequent marriage to Princess Chitrangada. The epic also mentions the metamorphosis of the princess from a warrior-like male personality into a soft, feminine woman learning the arts of dancing and music to win Arjuna's love.

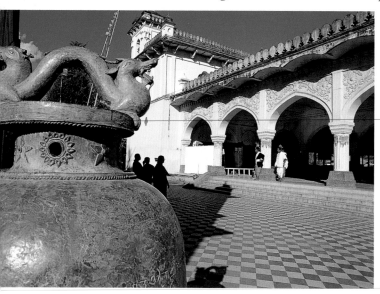

Nature-worship lies at the root of Manipur's traditional dances. Recognising the life-giving power of the cosmos and paying homage to the symbols of that power the ancient rituals are performed through dancing and singing and divining the mood of powers-to-be which are propitiated by the priests called Maiba. While the male priest, Maiba, involves himself in preparation and performance of the elaborate and lengthy rituals, the Maibi, comprising both the female and the male, also from priestly families, translates the creation of myths through dance and songs. Then the body moves in figures of eight in a continuum of flow of energy in many different patterns in space. The footfalls are petal-soft, the hands open and close with lotus movements and the fingers flutter like petals. Supple wrists play a very important role in Manipuri's *lasya* mode, i.e. the graceful feminine form.

PAGE 73
'Flowers'

ABOVE
Courtyard of Govindji temple in Imphal, Manipur. Even today every festival is celebrated here with rituals, music and dance

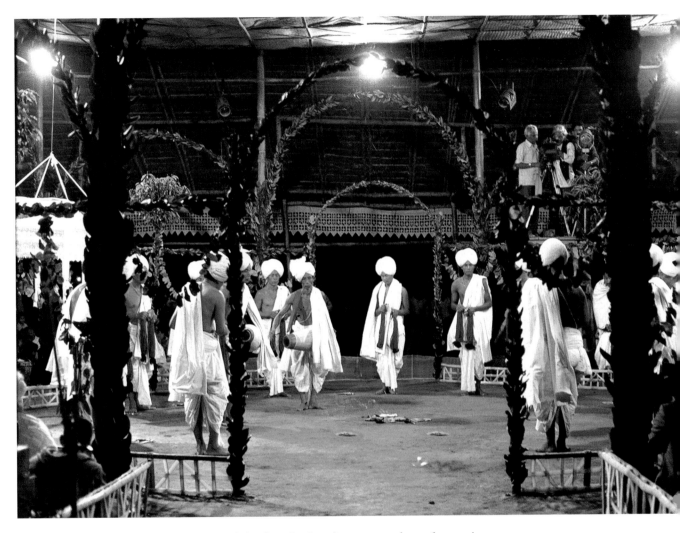

Clad in a hand-woven colourful *phanek* closely wrapped at the waist, somewhat like the *lungi*, and a tight blouse and gossamer white scarf wrapped around the torso, the Maibi woman recreates the process of creation of the world in which the earth and sky, the Sun and moon, the clouds and thunder, the rock and tree, the fruit and flower and ancestors — everything is offered for worship as being representative

ABOVE
Musicians with big cymbals and percussion doing Nata-Sankirtana in praise of Krishna inside the Govindji temple

agents of divine Nature. Snake-worship also has an important place in rituals and festivals and in dance choreography. Snakes separately or intertwined are depicted in hundreds of different patterns called *pafal*, i.e. the *mandala*. Even processions and groups of priests, dancers, musicians and devotees move in *pafal's* geometric patterns. The songs are accompanied by playing on *pena,* a small stringed instrument. One of the biggest festivals is Lai Haraoba for worship of god celebrated around the full-moon day at the beginning of summer. Legends about ancestors of indigenous Meitei people are enacted on special occasions.

In AD 1764, King Bhagyachandra of Manipur had a dream in which Krishna appeared and asked that his idol should be worshipped. The king forgot to fulfil his promise. One day a Naga (tribe) man came to the king and reminded him about the promised idol. A repentant king immediately ordered a beautiful idol to be carved out from the trunk of a sturdy jackfruit tree and installed it with pomp and ceremony in the Sri Govindji temple. Thus began the second phase of Manipuri culture when the cult of Vishnu-Krishna was introduced. This particular sect follows the Gaudiya Vaishnavism where Krishna is worshipped with his beloved Radha, who was already a married woman according to popular legend. At another level, Radha is understood to represent Krishna's divine energies without which he would be powerless. It is also a balancing of *yin* and *yang*, male and female elements of creation, where any imbalance would result in chaos and destruction.

Govinda is one of the many names of Krishna/Vishnu. Govinda literally means one 'who is light', knows the nature of light and is illumined by the knowledge of enlightenment. The king designed Sri Govindji's outfits and jewellery himself from whatever he remembered of his vision of Krishna in the dream. He also asked his favourite daughter, Princess Bimbavati Manjari, to enact the role of Radha in the first choreography of *Maha Raas* in Manipuri tradition and which he offered to Sri Govindji in the temple.

RIGHT
Krishna dancing with beloved Radha and her milkmaid friends occupies a major place in the repertory of Manipuri. It is called Raas Leela

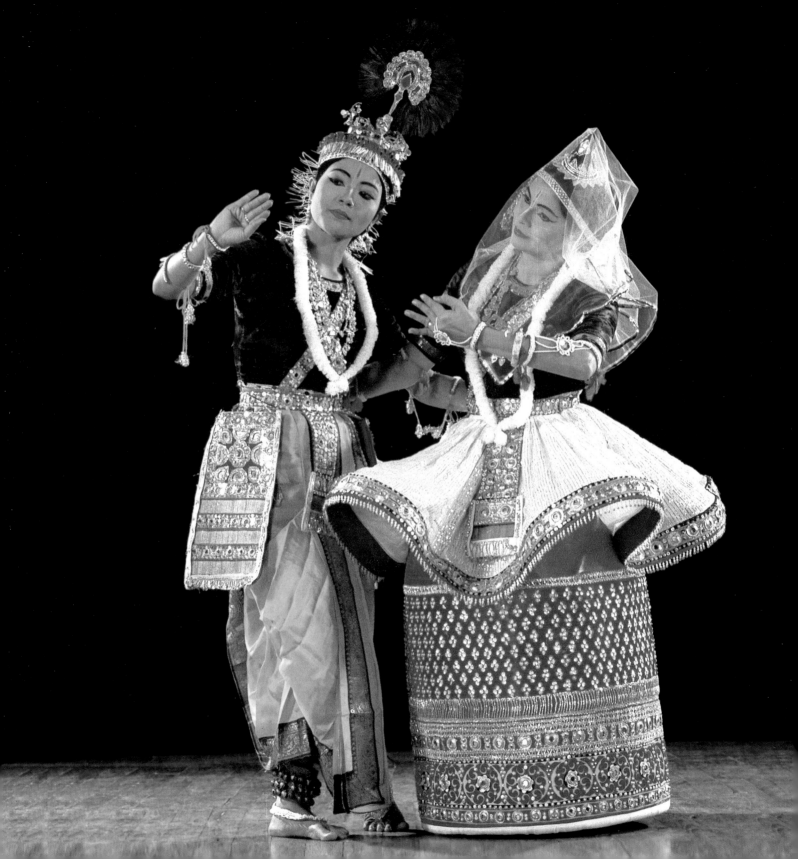

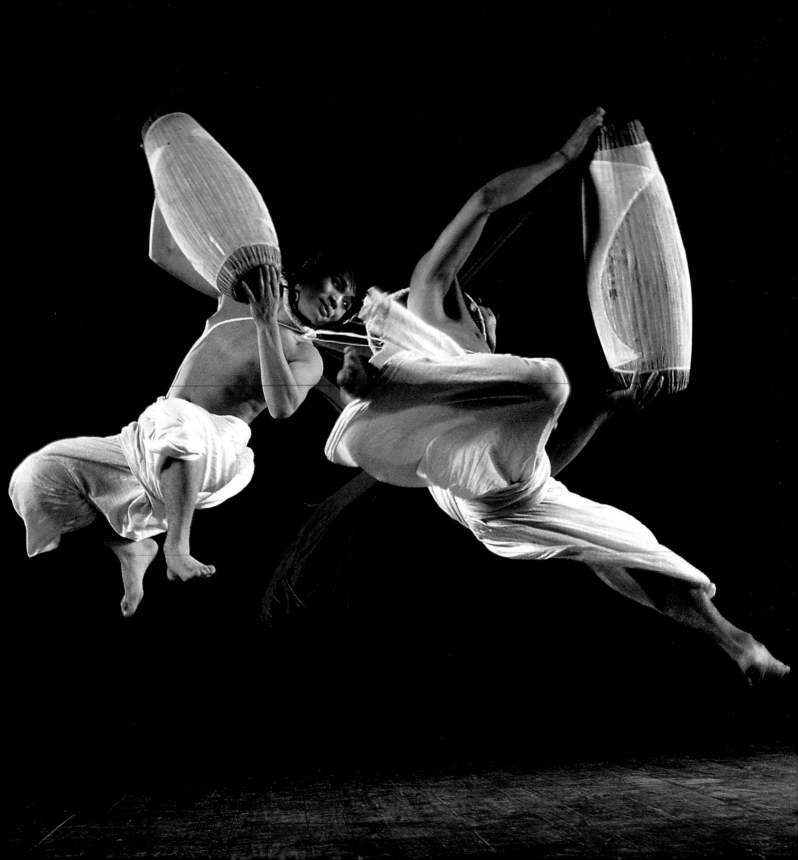

Four more varieties of *ras* dance choreographies emerged thereafter — Vasant Ras danced at spring-time; Kunja Ras where Krishna, Radha and her friends (*sakhi*) participate; Gopa Ras in which episodes from Krishna's childhood including his friendship with the innocent cowherds of Vraja are enacted; and Nitya Ras which may be performed on any occasion, any day. Yet there is a known system and order in which these are to be performed and in Manipur even a layman would not dare to violate it.

The two elements of masculine and feminine modes of dancing are clearly etched in the Manipuri technique. For example, in the masculine *tandava* mode, the male dancer pirouettes in spirals in space or on knees on the ground. The male dancer has many occasions to lift the leg high by lifting the knee. The female dancer in the *lasya* mode does not have this facility. Her *phanek* encasing her legs allows her to only slightly bend the knees in an *abhang* (slight flexion of knee) posture. A special composition which spells out the grammar and technique of Manipuri dance is called *bhangi pareng* which consists of a series of movements in both the male and female modes. It is like a dictionary of Manipuri dance technique from which teachers and choreographers draw out the material they need even today.

The costume for *ras* is very different from that of the Lai Haraoba. Here Krishna is usually danced by a young, agile boy, not older than 12 years of age. The men wear *dhoti* (unstitched) cloth tightly wrapped around each leg separately with the remaining cloth pleated like a folded fan in the front. Krishna always wears a yellow *dhoti* and jewellery of gold, beads, sequins, and peacock feathers. The women wear *polloi*, box-like skirts in bright greens and reds on which silver and gold sequins are stitched. The lower half of this skirt is rendered stiff with wires so that it does not swirl. Another shorter skirt in white tissue and bordered with mirrors and sequins is worn atop the box-skirt in curling folds. A tight, velvet, sequin-worked bodice, a white tissue scarf draped over a cone on the head and many ornaments and belts create a dazzling effect.

LEFT
Pung-cholam *(dance)*
with wild yet
controlled leaps and
jumps while playing
on the drum

The third element is the *nata sankeertana* which literally means 'singing praise through dance and music'. This is where the famous drum-dancers who leap, swirl and rotate with unimaginable dexterity while producing complex rhythmic patterns on the *mardal* (drum made of baked mud) are seen almost at every festival and event in India and abroad. Clad in simple white muslim *dhotis* and white turbans, they show breathtaking skill and virtuosity in managing the large drum slung from their lean but muscular shoulder along with choreographed walks and pirouettes in air and on the floor. This is called *pung-cholom* (playing on the *mardal* 'drum' called *pung* in Manipur). There are also *manjira* (cymbals) and *kartal* (palms of hands) with softer movements. *Pung-cholom* is always performed by male dancers while the other two include female dancers.

The fourth element of Manipuri dance technique is derived from the martial arts, *Thang-ta*. Techniques of attack, parry, re-group, etc. are instilled in the menfolk of Manipur who demonstrate excellent suppleness, agility and manoeuvres with real sword, lance, mace, stick, dagger and whatever else that can be used in warfare. These men are also excellent horsemen. The dance derives many movements from observing such manoeuvres.

The textual material for Manipuri dance today is taken from the *Gita Govinda, Anand Vrindavan Champoo, Govind Sangeet Leela-mritan* and other Vaishnavite works. The Lai Haraoba songs, of course, use the ancient language of the Meitei people. Compositions preserved through oral traditions too are an integral part of the pool of material used for Manipuri dance which, because of its geographical distance from other parts of India and the religious fervour of the people, promises to retain its character and identity for a long time to come.

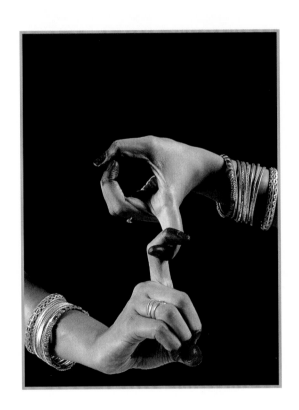

Kuchipudi

Kuchelapuram is a small village in Andhra Pradesh. The descendants of 300 Brahmin families live here to continue a tradition that dictates that only men may dance. The village and the land are gifts from the Nawab of Golconda, in 1675, after witnessing a performance of a Kuchipudi dance-drama by migrant Brahmins. The tradition of *natya* using poetry, drama, dance and music have a long history in the regions now known as Tamil Nadu, Andhra Pradesh and Karnataka, the thematic content always being based on a glorified devotion to god-*bhakti,* therefore the participants came to be known as *bhaktas* while the form is called the Bhagvat Mela Natakam.

A great devotee of Vishnu, Siddhendra *yogi* had a dream in which he witnessed the enchanting vision of Lord Krishna with his two favourite consorts, Rukmini and Satyabhama. The dream unfolded the story of the *parijata,* the heavenly tree, which was coveted by both the wise and stately Rukmini and the beautiful, haughty Satayabhama, following an altercation inspired by the ever-present and mischievous sage, Narada. Krishna sought to placate his queens by setting off heavenwards to obtain the tree for his palace.

Overcome with joy and devotion, Siddhendra *yogi* began a search for dancers and actors who would enact this play of his dream. He found suitable young men among the Brahmin families of Kuchelapuram. It was the enactment of this dream-vision on stage that pleased the Nawab of Golconda. Since then, every Brahmin family of the village ritually offers at least one male member to be trained as an actor-dancer. The name of the village changed to Kuchipudi as time passed and its dance-drama also acquired this name. Today it has retained the name and form with its earthy flavour and seductive body language.

The families initiated into this art were given a thorough training in various aspects of *Naya Shastra*. A thorough training in dance, singing, speech, rhetoric, Sanskrit and Telugu poetry was required before the dancer

PAGE 81
'Quarrel, enmity,
opposition'

RIGHT
Scene from a dance-
drama, Srinivasa
Kalyanam, on the
theme of marriage of
the Divine pair,
Vishnu and
Padmavati
- Disciples of Shobha
Naidu

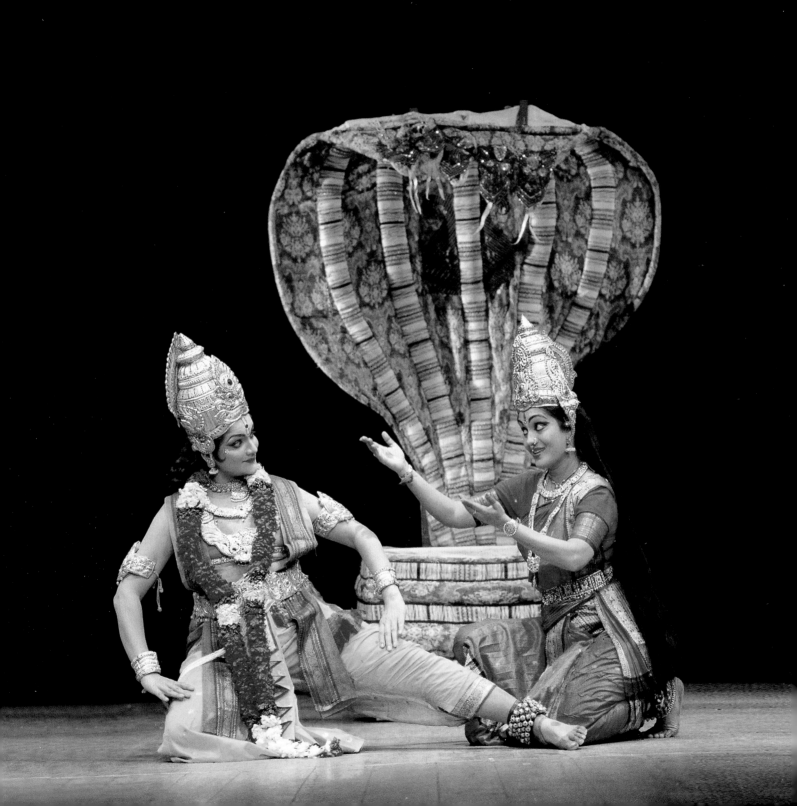

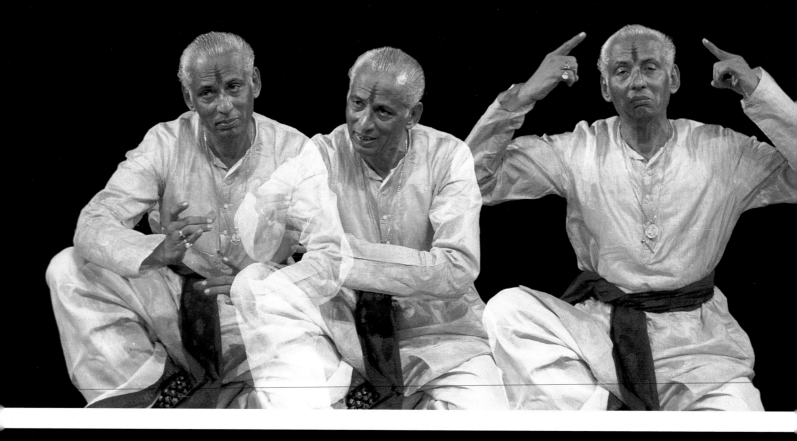
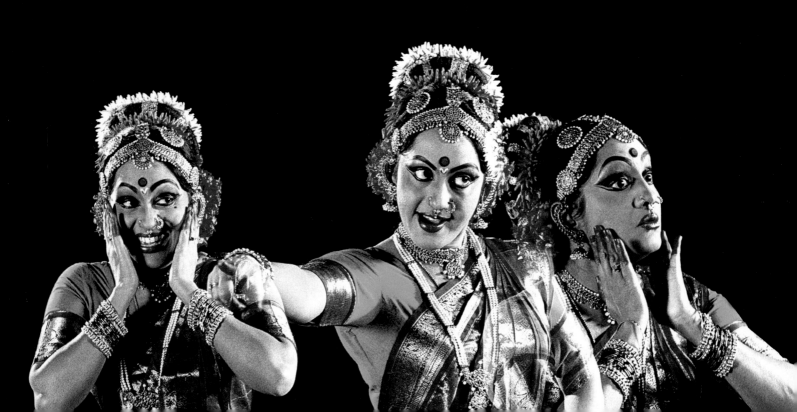

was allowed on the stage even in a small role. Fortunately, this continues till today, keeping alive the mainstream of aesthetic understanding of Indian culture without which no art form can flourish, especially in India. The technique of Kuchipudi is *natya*, which includes the twin arts of dance and music besides acting. The acting is of two kinds — one where the *sutradhar* (narrator) dialogues with the characters, using speech as an instrument of narration. Naturally, therefore, the accompanying gestures and expressions are direct and simple. The other kind of acting involves the dancer-actors performing on music, using the prescribed hand gestures, facial expressions and footwork.

Let us consider the important differences in the styles of presentation of a particular theme, event or episode. There are two modes — one is *natyadharmi* and the other is *lokdharmi*. The first interprets the theme purely with the help of systematised and codified gestures, stances and expressions. The second takes recourse to popular devices like theatrical movements, expressions and realistic costumes, make-up and bearing. For example, in the *natyadharmi* presentation, the demon Ravana is depicted with hand gestures, showing the number 10 (for symbolically showing intellect and power superior to a single person), one hand in *shakatasya*, held near the face (denoting fangs) and the other hand tracing the round outline of the face, *alla padma* (gestures) to denote heads, thus completing the depiction of the 10-headed demon. In the *lokdharmi* representation, these and other such characteristics of Ravana are used wherever the context allows, but the character of Ravana is firmly fixed by planting a huge crown and nine, painted heads on the shoulder of the dancer who then continues being Ravana rather than characterising him.

This differentiation is naturally most noticeable in the solo styles vis-a-vis dance-dramas styles. Given below is a description of one of the most popular dance-drama narratives.

Usha is the beautiful daughter of the mighty king Banasur of Kamarupa who ruled in the region now called Assam. One morning Usha awoke from

ABOVE LEFT
Various moods from a story - Vempati Chinna Satyam

BELOW LEFT
Aspects of a woman in love - Shobha Naidu

her sleep, distressed and disturbed. She confided her dream to her dearest friend Chitralekha. She had seen a most handsome man and had fallen in love with him. Her condition was now so hopeless that unless she was helped, she would surely die. Chitralekha set to work immediately. She was endowed with a rare gift — that of drawing accurate portraits from scratchy descriptions. Haltingly, Usha described her dream-man. Chitralekha fetched her easel and paints and produced one portrait after another, before painting a portrait of the ruler of Dwarka, Shri Krishna Vasudeva. Usha noted the resemblance and begged Chitralekha to paint his family members as well. Chitralekha then drew Pradyumna, son of Shri Krishna. Usha grew more excited. Suddenly she grew quiet and bashful as the portrait emerged. When Chitralekha looked up, she knew she had hit the right target and her joy knew no bounds. She cajoled Chitralekha to make him available to her. Chitralekha complied. Using her divine gift she flew to Dwarka and brought back a sleeping Anirudhha on bed. The episode comes to its natural conclusion with their happy union.

Let me describe the stage presentation of the play. After the ceremonial *ranga puja* (worship offered to the performance arena) the curtain-bearers take up positions behind which Princess Usha performs her salutations to the gods and gurus. At the right moment, the curtain is lowered to reveal Usha, young and innocent, playful and vivacious. She is shown whiling away the hours in the company of her friends, playing on instruments, making garlands, teasing and playing. At the end of the revelry, which is danced with a fine feminine touch, the chief dancer, Vedantam, in the role of Usha, takes up the sleeping posture. The accompanying music symbolises the passage of time. The sequence in which Usha is shown suddenly awake but dreamy-eyed, happy but distressed, is mimed in the inimitable style of a real 16-year old girl. The confession of the dream and Chitralekha's promise to help her concludes the sequence. In sharp contrast to the refined, delicate and subtle portrayal of Usha, two characters stride on to the stage, dressed as the king

RIGHT
A group choreography (left to right) – Radha, Yamini, Bhavana and Kaushalya Reddy with Raja Reddy seated in centre

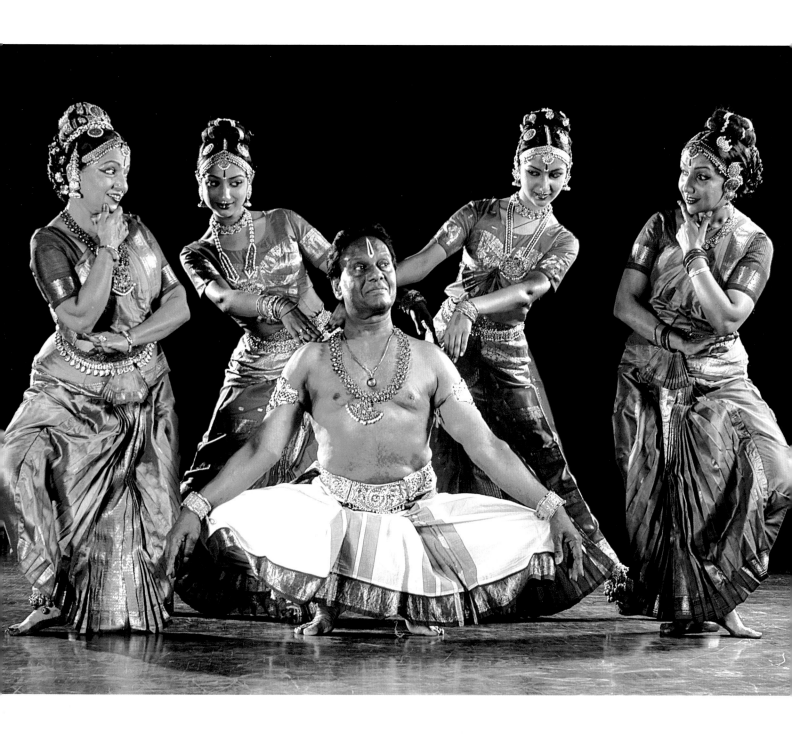

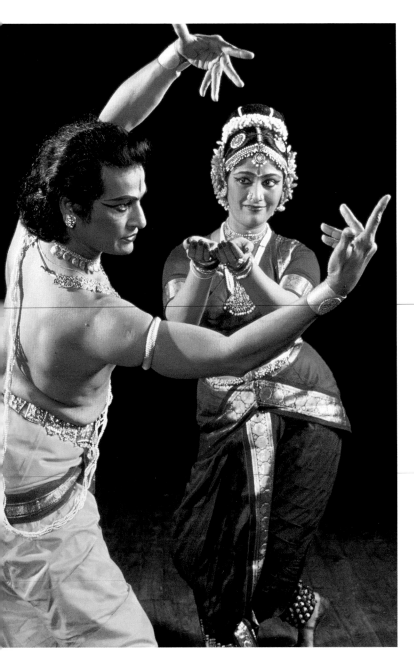

and his minister. While Usha's costume is simple and conforms to the precept of *natyadharmi* mode, the two men are shown with crowns and robes, swords hanging from their sashes and big moustaches covering half their faces. They engage in a dialogue punctuated by short songs, gesticulating freely, which makes for the *lokadharmi* mode of acting. The chief musician, dressed as the *sutradhar*, is also a part of the scene.

From this populistic interjection, once again the play reverts to the *natyadharmi*, showing Usha in earnest conversation with her friend. Through gestures, measured steps and facial expressions that bespeak a deep understanding of the character and the tenets that govern the characterisation, and combined with a fine restraint, Usha, the young princess in love, is brought alive. When Chitralekha begins to draw the dream-man, the *lokadharmi* again establishes itself because under the strict *natyadharmi* rules, the portraits, the easel and the act of painting would all be shown through gestures with appropriate responses on the face. Here instead, actual pictures are being shown one by one and rejected quickly.

Thereafter the scene shows Anirudhha, recumbent on his bed, painted blue from top to toes, signifying his family ties with Shri Krishna. Now he is in Usha's chamber. Beginning with Usha's feigned reluctance to even look at her lover, the dancer-actor traverses a vast range of conflicting emotions, using every possible mood, sentiment, shading, stance, posture, gesture and glance to fuel the sentiment *sringara* (love). Giving in to Chitralekha's entreaties and following her ardent desire, Usha is portrayed as circumambulating the bed

of the sleeping Aniruddha, peeping shyly, stealing glances, resenting her own bashfulness and using flower petals as a means of establishing contact gently. The evocation of the mood takes up almost half an hour before Anirudhha is awakened. With alternating suggestions of happiness and shy ness — a slightly fearful Usha and a proud and wondrous Anirudhha — the dance-drama is brought to an end. As might have been apparent from this description, it is a happy blend of the two modes of presentation that enhance its dramatic value without detracting from the subtle nuances of acting.

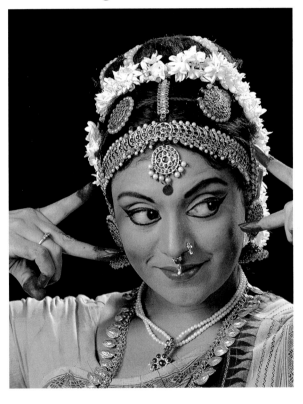

The flow of the narrative element in Kuchipudi is punctuated by pieces of pure dance, performed to the accompaniment of *shollu kattu* of short or long duration, depending on the situation and character. At first glance, the pure dance in Kuchpudi might appear very similar to Bharatanatyam, but on closer examination one notices the typical thrusts, extensions, dancing on toes and sequences that begin just after the beat, and which are typical of Kuchipudi. Also, the body is allowed to sway more languorously and freely than is ever possible in Bharatanatyam.

Some of the well-loved and oft-repeated dance-dramas in Kuchipudi are *Bhama Kalapam* taken from the famous work *Parijata Paharana* by Siddhendra Yogi, *Golla Kalapam* by Ramayya Shastri, the *Krishna Lila Tarangini* by Tirtha Narayana Yati, the *Gita Govinda* of Jaidev, the Telugu songs of Kshetrayya and the *Kritis* by Thyagaraja. Dance-dramas are performed regularly in Kuchipudi and the surrounding villages, especially on festival days.

As was seen in the traditional dance-drama, actor-dancers wear costumes and make-up suitable to the character. The solo Kuchipudi dancer wears a costume similar to that in Bharatanatyam. A red sari tied slightly higher than normal, or a stitched costume of rich material, opens into an ankle-length fan in front and a pleated border tucked at the back. The hair is pleated in a long braid decorated with flowers and a bejewelled hair-piece called *rakhudi*. There is an interesting legend about the special *jadai* (head ornament) worn by Satyabhama in the dance-drama *Bhama Kalapam*. The ornament contains the Sun and the moon, the 27 *nakshatras* (constellations), the mighty hooded serpent, parrots and floral motifs representing creation or *prakriti* (Nature), which is represented by Satayabhama. Traditionally this ornament had been ceremonially presented to the best dancer in the portrayal of Satyabhama. Even the way of showing off this oranament is special. At the time of the entrance of Satyabhama, the curtain is brought forward as usual with Satyabhama walking behind it. The braid is thrown over the curtain in full view of the audience. The braid acquires a significance all its own while Satyabhama dances her initial salutations behind the curtain. The flaunting of the braid which is a challenge to spectators, is symbolic of Satyabhama's supremacy as a dancer, a woman and the favourite of Krishna.

The orchestra in Kuchipudi comprises the guru who also acts as the *sutradhar,* cymbals in hand and is responsible for the flow of the performance. A vocalist, a *mridangam* player accompanied by flute and violin players complete the ensemble.

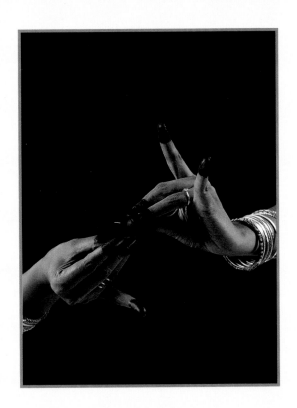

Sattriya

The *namghars* in Assam, in the north-east region of India, are temples not unlike some early temples in Japan. At the ancient temple of Itsukushima, the altar in the sanctum sanctorum has only two objects — a mirror and a sword. Rest of the temple consists of a large hall and smaller spaces for holding ritual ceremonies or for observing meditative silence.

The place of worship is called *namghar* in the village but in the monastery the name changes to *kirtanghar*, meaning 'the place for singing praises and taking Lord's name'. The altar has a beautifully carved and painted wooden object with seven levels to denote the seven heavens of Vishnu or *sapta vaikuntha* on which is placed the *Srimad Bhagawad*, the ancient text composed by sage Veda Vyasa, to depict the life and deeds of Shri Krishna who is synonymous with Vishnu, the presiding deity at all the *sattras*. The offerings of food, sweets, fruits, etc. are made in a tall brass vessel called *sarai* in Tamil or mouth-fresheners are kept in a smaller one made of bell-metal and called *bota*. An intricately woven long piece of cloth, silk or fine cotton, with the Lord's name, is draped behind the altar. It is *gohain gamocha* and is specially woven for this purpose but unlike those found in the market.

Among the *sattra*, two ways of living are allowed. In some only celibate monks live forming a family bond with the older monks. Here the *kirtanghar* is at the centre of the *sattra* while the monks live on the four sides of the central hall. In the second kind, monks are allowed to marry and live with their families in the *sattra*. The head of the monastery, known as *sattradhikari*, literally meaning 'authority of the monastery', looks after the administration and welfare of the place. His house may become the focal point for all activities.

Some monasteries form a group adhering to one main *sattra*, e.g. *kamalabari* which has a group of six or seven monasteries of only celibate monks. This *sattra* is particularly famous for a festival lasting four days during which the monks perform the rarely seen compositions of dance and music and dance-dramas otherwise poor materially. Such *sattras* house great

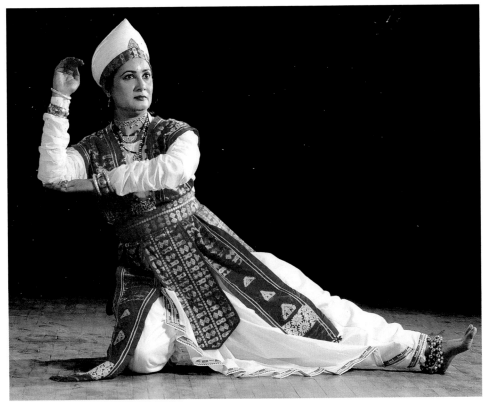

artistic treasures. During the festivals such as this, singing of *kirtans* constitutes the main activity. Sometimes as many as 14 sessions of singing the Lord's name are organised. There are also those praising the names of Sankaradeva who introduced Vaishnavism to Assam, his chief disciple Madhav Deo and Padmata, who was sent in place of Madhav Deo to propagate Vaishnavism to far off places. For that reason *Padmata* (*Ata* meaning 'father') came to be called Badula meaning "in place of...."

Sattra is a monastery where young boys are trained in the arts of dance, music and acting along with regular spiritual meditation. Respectfully called Srimant Sanskar Deo or Mahapurusha Sanskar Deo (1449-1568), this saintly scholar of Sanskrit introduced a new concept in devotional practice of the *sattra*. It was founded as an institution for the pursuit and preservation of

ABOVE
'The raised hood of a cobra' - Sharodi Saikia

Classical Dances   93

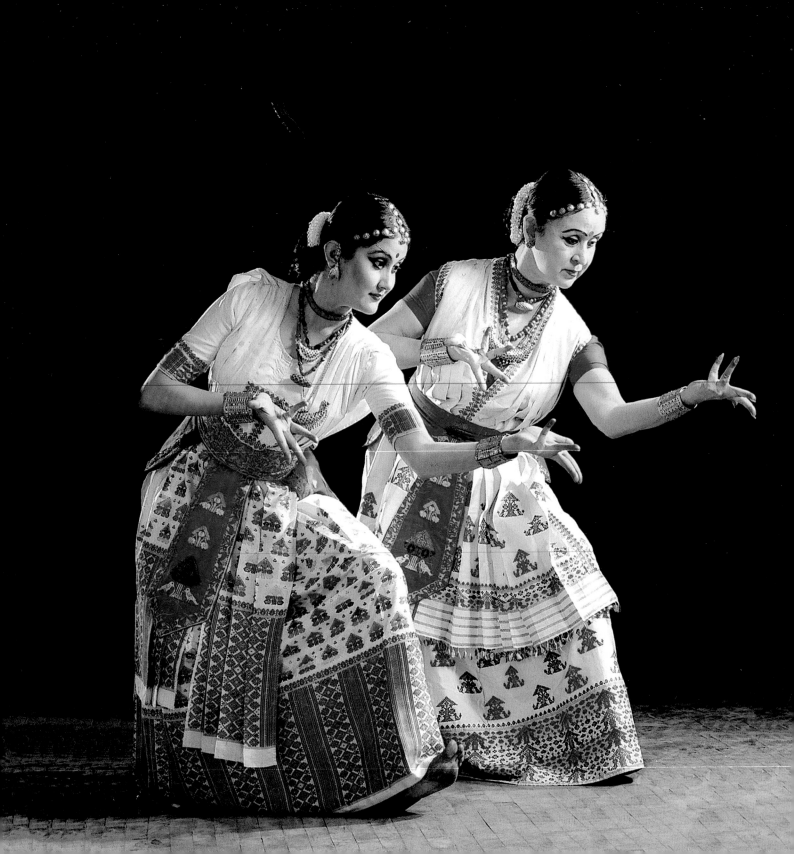

bhakti to Lord Vishnu and total devotion and faith in the Lord. Interestingly this also brought about co-mingling of diverse art forms indigenous to the land but not merely as an artistic pursuit. The devices of dance, music and drama were used for propagation. The faith in a few *sattras* meant that to become celibate monks, young boys between the age of five to seven years are given rigorous training in various aspects of *sattra* discipline and learning, including the performing arts. Titles of *gayan* (singer) and *bayan* (player) are conferred on those who after years of training under various senior teachers show merit and proficiency. The name of the dance style emanating from the *sattra* came to be known as Sattriya.

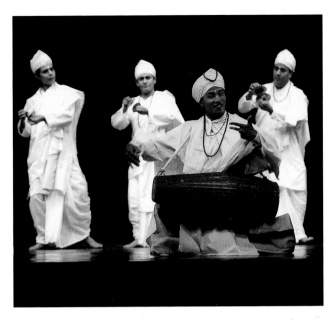

Although today female dancers have taken to this in a large number, as mentioned earlier only male monks used to dance. The grammar of this dance style as seen today comprises three elements or techniques used in the gymnasium and called *maati akhara, ankiya nat* and *oja palli*. *Maati akhara* consists of 64 movements of dance that eschews story-telling or expressional content. Therefore there are 64 units of pure dance among which some denote male vigour, others the female grace and the third may look neutral.

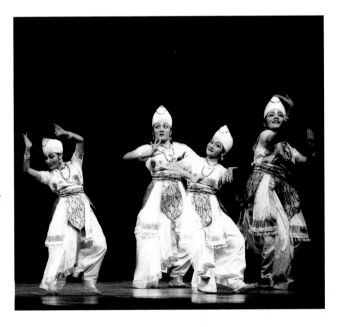

Culling from the existent indigenous performing art traditions, Sankara-deva drew inspiration from the semi-dramatic form of *oja pali*. It is basically choral singing, the group consisting of the *oja* (master) and the *palis* (assistants). The group has five to six persons parallel to the *pala* of Orissa and the *oja* recites verses from a scriptural text, at times on a specific theme. The recitation is visually exacted through hand gestures and body movements. The accompanists keep time on the cymbals while repeating the lines of the text.

The Sattriya dance technique today underlines *bhakti* (devotion) as the main flavour of the style. Surprisingly, the entire range of lyrics and texts used for dance has no mention of Radha, the beloved *gopi* of Krishna, possibly because it would have meant condoning the emotion of love between man and woman and called *sringara rasa* in classic texts. Sankaradeva ignored Radha in preference to *gopis* — a group of women who pined for, loved and worshipped Sri Krishna. This is a major point of departure from all the other dance styles of India.

The technique shows a body that arches and curves without showing straight lines, square or triangular postures. The upper torso moves independently of the lower body, similar to the *taranga* movement in Odissi. The body dips and rises in a bobbing continuum giving an illusion of weightlessness. Many ways of walk, jump, sit and pirouette which are typical to Sattriya have developed, imparting it a flavour and form all its own.

Costumes are made from Assamese silk. *Mekhla chadar* and *gamocha* are in cotton. Colours like white and red are prominent as is the ubiquitous sandalwood mark on the forehead.

PAGE 94
A harmorious stance typical of Sattriya dance
- Indira P.P.Bora and Menaka

PAGE 95
'Gayan-bayan' means singing and playing on percussion instruments. This is usually performed at the beginning of a recital
- Ghanakant Bora and group

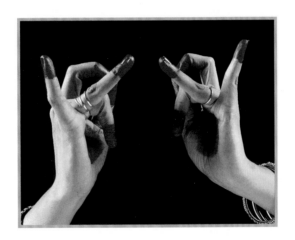

Mohiniattam

This dance style from Kerala in South India derives its name from two words — *mohini* meaning 'enchantress' and *attam* meaning 'dance'. The grand dance-theatre of Kerala called Kathakali made strenuous and strong demands on the body and which could be answered only by the male dancers. So, a graceful form of dance more suited to the female body gradually took form based on the existing dances performed during marriages, festivals and other social occasions. The strong influence of the *Natya Shastra* (the compendium on acting, dance and music) already rooted in Kerala provided the grammar and structure to formulate this style. As its *raison d'etre*, it derived inspiration from the ancient legend of *samundra manthan* (churning of the Milky Ocean). Putting aside their habitual enmity, the gods and anti-gods or demons decided to launch a joint project — the search for ambrosia, the elixir of immortality. They had heard it being said that it could be found at the bottom of the Milky Ocean. So planting the high mountain, Mandara, as the churning rod and twining the sinuous serpent Vasuki around it, they set to work. After a routine squabble on who would hold the either ends of the serpent, the gods wisely let the anti-gods hold on to the venom-spewing head while holding the tail end themselves. At a signal, the churning of the ocean began. One by one, 12 jewel-like items surfaced. Among them were the moon, the conch, the tree of life, a wish-fulfilling cow, four celestial dancers, a goddess of prosperity, king of elephants, the fastest horse, the divine healer, a dazzling jewel, a mighty bow and a garland of victory. Suddenly the waters turned dark blue and black. Poisonous fumes engulfed the cosmic breath. Gods and anti-gods screamed for help because the all-consuming *halahala* (poison) had begun to emerge. Together they prayed and Shiva appeared to rescue the creation by drinking up the poison and holding it in his throat. Because of this, the legend says, Shiva's throat turned blue giving him the title of Neelakanth. Once this calamity was over, both parties set to work with redoubled zeal. Their reward — a golden pot containing *amrita* (ambrosia)

PAGE 97
'A dialogue of birds'

RIGHT
Depicting something beautiful through the glance, smile and hand gestures
- Bharati Shivaji

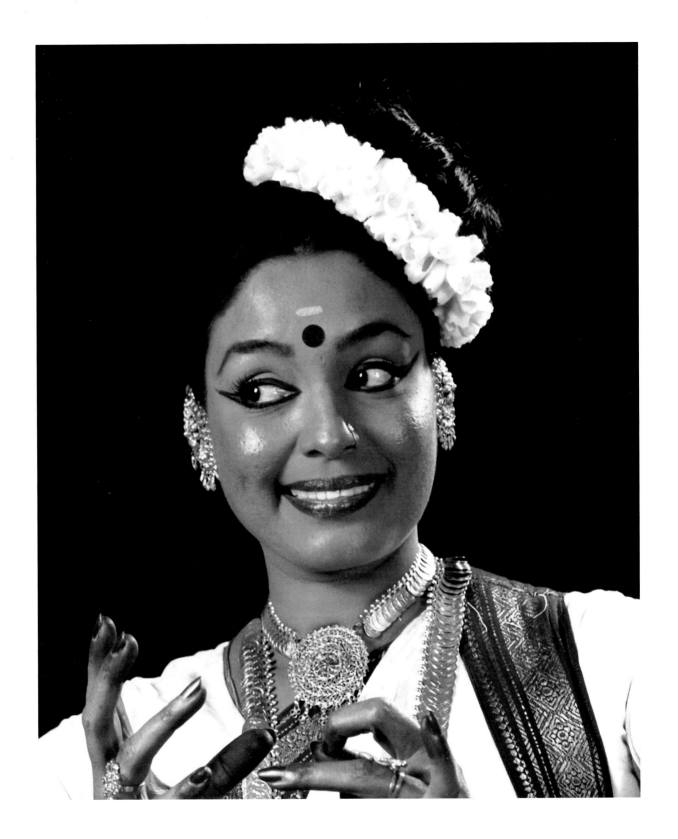

bobbed up. In a trice it was snatched away by the ever-vigilant anti-gods. This was a warning bell for the gods because if the anti-gods were to drink it and become immortal, all would be destroyed except for the anti-gods. The gods prayed to Vishnu, who was known for amending situations created by Brahma or Shiva. At the very moment soft cool breeze carrying the heady aroma of a beautiful woman wafted in the air and there came and stood Vishnu in the form of a bewitching beauty. The anti-gods fell prey to the gorgeous female and asked her to resolve their dilemma of rank and status. Even the gods staked their claim to the ambrosia. Mohini accepted to become the arbiter and asked them to sit down facing each other to facilitate distribution of *amrita*.

Mohini began her graceful dance of enchantment and tricked the gods into receiving the elixir while the anti-gods could only look on helplessly. The gods, now empowered with *amrita,* regrouped and fought off the anti-gods by pushing them back to where they had come from.

A second legend refers to Mohini-Vishnu in connection with the arrogant and powerful king, Bhasmasura who won his title as a boon-giver by Shiva whereby he could reduce anything to ash by merely placing his hand on it. This was a terrible situation where the arrogant and power-hungry demonic king could destroy the world. Once again on hearing the pleas of frightened gods, Vishnu appeared as Mohini, the bewitching beauty. She agreed to marry on the condition that the king would defeat her in a dance duel. Mohini danced many patterns which the enchanted king imitated easily. As the tempo of dancing increased, Mohini performed a movement placing her hand on her head. The king followed suit and no sooner did he place his hand on his head than he was reduced to a pile of ash. Once again Mohini saved creation from destruction.

Therefore a dance form, which derives its inspiration and name from such a concept, has to contain soft, bewitching movements. The waist is the fulcrum on which the upper and lower body twists and turns in gentle

RIGHT
A lovelorn heroine stringing flowers to offer the garland to her beloved
- Kanak Rele

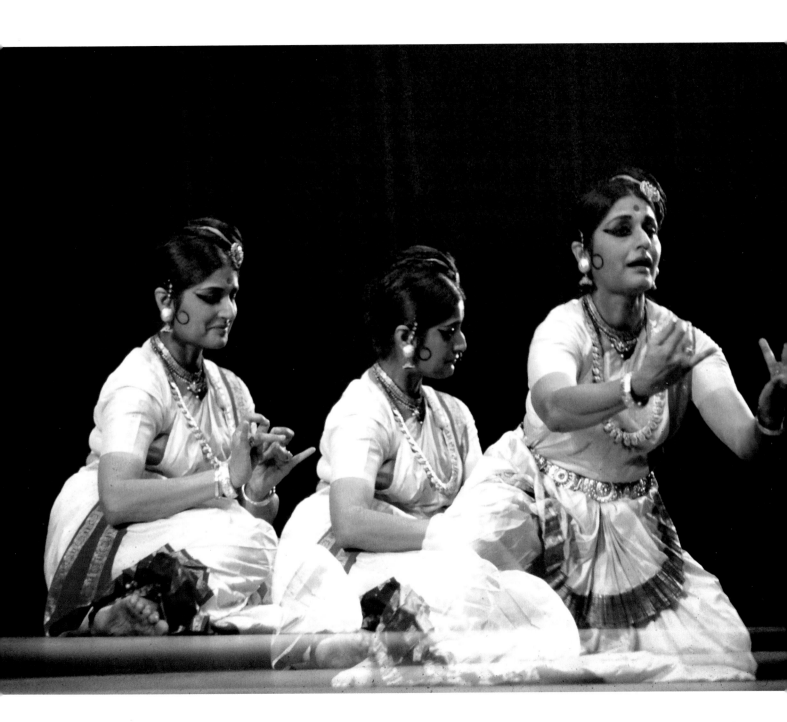

curving figures of eight or in a half-moon shape. The geometry of lines is supple yet soft. The footwork is rich yet delicately delineated. Although Kathakali is a sibling form, the movements of eyes and eyebrows are toned down from the accented, strong glances to soft, inviting ones. Hand gestures too speak of feminine grace and subtlety of expression.

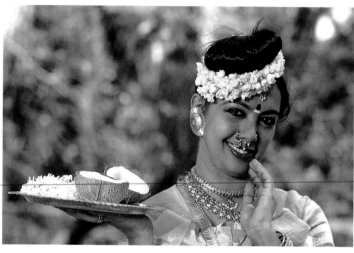

The costume is invariably in white, bordered with gold and draped in a way that allows plenty of space for leg extensions (never high but to the side). A huge fan-like effect is created in front by bunching and pleating the upper border of the sari at the waist. The hairstyle sports a big bun to the left side of the head, encircled by flowers and jewels. Simple but attractive gold, ruby and emerald jewellery is worn.

A typical system of music developed to accompany these dances, is called *sopana*. The ladder-like soft, entrancing dance movements, accompanied by music that ascends and descends on melodious notes in a prearranged pattern, seem to undulate and sway along with the body of the dancer.

This dance form reached its zenith in the early 19th century in the royal court of King Swathi Tirunal of Travancore in Kerala. He was a poet, writer, scholar, linguist and a great and informed patron of the arts.

Mohiniattam does not have a temple background but rather a social and secular one with inclination towards sentiments and emotions of love in all its glorious manifestations. A judicious use of beckoning eyes and fluttering eyebrows summon the viewer's attention at will, justifying the form as a dance of the enchantress. For this is a dance form for and by women only.

ABOVE
A Mohiniattam dancer in her typical make-up and costume

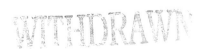